REVIEWS FOR

EAT SLEEP MOVE BREATHE

I love this book! If you asked me to take decades of experience working at the bleeding edge of human athletic performance and boil it to the most essential behaviors for long term, sustainable success, it would be this book! The trick to unlocking our incredibly robust and antifragile natures is to appreciate the way that the keystone behaviors in this book integrate into a cogent whole. Performing these "basics" well for the rest of your life will never get old or go out of style. The principles within these pages are the fundamentals of being a truly savage human.

—Dr. Kelly Starrett, DPT
Coach, Physio, Co-Founder of *The Ready State 2x NYT Best Selling Author.*

***

I found that this book, ***Eat Sleep Move Breathe***, was very well researched and written. The book is easy to read and to follow. I believe this book provides a well-rounded approach to gain and maintain great health.

—Dr. Harold J. Bowersox, D.O., M.B.A., M.S
Author of *"The Bowersox Protocol for Fibromyalgia and Chronic Fatigue."*

***

Eat Sleep Move Breathe is a wonderful introductory guide to living more fully. As basic global health has shifted over the past fifty years due to changes in our work environments, food supply, and traditional ways of living, each of the components the authors address is crucial for health and vitality. As experts in this field, the authors use wonderful stories to make the steps to wellness accessible and simple to implement. They cover the most important aspects of health, healing, and vitality; spending time with this book and implementing the recommendations will jump you from a wellness novice into a lifestyle deeply rooted in the transformation into health and vitality.

—Dr. Ann Marie Chiasson

Director of Fellowship in Integrative Medicine, Associate Clinical Professor of Medicine, *Andrew Weil Center for Integrative Medicine, University of Arizona, Tucson, Arizona.*

EAT

SLEEP

MOVE

BREATHE

A Beginner's Guide to Living A Healthy Lifestyle

Lars Thestrup, MD

Jennifer Pfleghaar, DO

Connor Martin

Published by KHARIS PUBLISHING, imprint of KHARIS
MEDIA LLC.

Copyright © 2020 Lars Thestrup, MD. Jenny Pfleghaar, DO.
Connor Martin

ISBN-13: 978-1-946277-78-7
ISBN-10: 1-946277-78-9

Library of Congress Control Number: 2020943682

All KHARIS PUBLISHING products are available at special
quantity discounts for bulk purchase for sales   promotions,
premiums, fund-raising, and educational needs.
For details, contact:

Kharis Media LLC
Tel: 1-479-599-8657
support@kharispublishing.com
www.kharispublishing.com

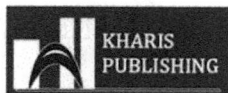

CONTENTS

INTRODUCTION

Back when humans made buildings from stone, the most important block they quarried was the cornerstone. This was the first stone set in the construction of the building. In fact, all other stones that came after would reference that foundational setting stone. That's what made them so vital. If your cornerstone was true, the building would be true.

When it comes to personal health, there seems to be a lot of shaky ground and a lot of crooked stones, so it's hard to know how to build a strong, healthy foundation. Within this book, we have developed four cornerstones for building a healthy lifestyle: diet, sleep, meditation, and exercise. If we can set each of these concepts as our cornerstones, we have a stable foundation for structuring our health.

So where did this idea come from?

With a combined 30 years of work experience in the emergency department and 10 years of personal training, we have each encountered many individuals with cases of chronic diseases like diabetes, hypertension (HTN), and coronary artery disease. Many of the diseases afflicting our clientele could have been prevented if only they had lived a healthier lifestyle. During this era of pandemics, there appears to be an even greater value in being healthy. Eliminating underlying medical conditions can improve outcomes, should you fall ill.

Not long ago, a young person in their early twenties visited the ER. They were morbidly obese with multiple health problems. They questioned, "Why do I have these problems? Why am I so obese?"

After asking several questions about their lifestyle, it was discovered that they ate fast food three times a day, slept four hours a night, had no time for themselves, and never exercised. Diet, sleep, meditation, exercise? Apparently, no one had ever told them about the importance of these behaviors. Sure, they had seen books on these topics, but they were too long and dense; they were overwhelming. This lack of basic facts is what gave birth to the concept of a beginner's guide, a quick and easily digestible manual that lays out the cornerstones of a healthy lifestyle.

Part of the beauty of this concept is simplicity. These four cornerstones all rely on each other to create a stable foundation. Without a healthy diet, your exercise performance suffers. Without exercise, your ability to get good, restful sleep is hindered. When you're sleep deprived, your mental health can be significantly affected. And when you're not thinking straight, you're more likely to make emotional decisions with your diet. Each one has a direct impact on the other. So, if we can get each cornerstone concept right, we can have a stronger body and a more stable mind.

You don't have to chisel out all four healthy concepts to be successful. Focusing your energy on just one, even in a simple and basic way, can have a profound impact on your health. You can improve your life in big ways by committing to a small change in behavior. Take it one day at a time. Gradually ease into the concept that most interests you. Over time you will find yourself eating healthier, sleeping better, focusing on your mental well-being, and even moving and exercising more. It's not a diet or fad, and it's not a program to follow. Think of it as a process, a natural progression. Just make yourself these two promises:

1. I will start by making one small change

2. I will not be too hard on myself

After all, as the old adage goes: *Rome wasn't built in a day.* Rather, it was built one stone at a time. With these four cornerstones of health, you'll be on your way to building a better you. Any progress on any of these four cornerstones is a step in the right direction.

EAT

THE CAUSE AND THE CURE

Amy was a young woman that came in frequently
to the ER where I worked. So frequently in fact,
that I probably saw her more often than her primary care doctor.

She was in her twenties though not in good health. While
she could function in her daily activities, Amy wasn't feeling
great physically or mentally. She was overweight. Her joints
ached. She was plagued with chronic belly pain and yeast
infections. Amy also suffered from depression. She was exhausted and worn out from constant physical and mental
struggles.

Most of her visits to the ER were related to chronic
abdominal pain, which often resulted in a CT scan. Owing
to the frequency of these scans, her risk of radiation induced
cancer was now increasing. During one of her visits, we
discussed the frequent scans as yet another risk factor for

her. Amy's challenges felt endless.

It became clear that Amy didn't need another CT scan; she needed information about how to develop a healthier diet. We discussed making changes to her diet: eliminating soda, chips, and fast food. I encouraged her to keep a food diary to better understand triggers for her acid reflux. These simple steps and the realization that she could have some control over her symptoms was the "Aha" moment for her.

By making a basic switch, such as replacing processed foods with fresh fruit and vegetables, Amy found herself on a completely different path. It's a simple prescription for health, yet nutrition is not widely known or considered "medicine" in its own right. A small amount of information can make a huge difference in helping us know how to start making changes. Further, we can really understand why these food choices matter to our health, and thus provide us with the motivation to change.

Amy wasn't the first (or the last) patient I would see in the ER with nutrition as both the cause and the cure of their disease.

LET'S BEGIN

We have all heard this saying before: *You are what you eat.* What you put into your body can make a difference in how you look, how you feel, and how you behave. Not only is food used for energy, but the correct food can help prevent cancer, decrease depression, help with PMS, and even prevent you from getting sick.

Additionally, food can provide us with important vitamins, minerals, and phytonutrients. These include indole-3-carbinol and lignans, all of which help prevent certain cancers. Broccoli and Brussels sprouts are examples of vegetables containing indole-3-carbinol. Lignans are found in flaxseeds, soybeans, and other seeds. Flavonoids, found in strawberries, spinach, and much more, are great as anti-inflammatory foods.[i] Eating the right foods can help us prevent cancer, battle inflammation which can result in damage to healthy tissues and organs, and provide ourselves with natural vitamins.

We often use the word "diet" when what we really mean is a healthy food lifestyle. The lifestyle that I'm referring to is one that includes eating whole foods instead of processed foods, eating food with a variety of colors, eating seasonal foods, buying fresh food at farmers markets, cooking at home, and minimizing empty calories. Examples of empty calories are: soda, slushies, cookies, candy, potato chips, and ice cream. Nutrient-dense foods include broccoli, salmon, spinach, nuts, and strawberries.

Have you ever noticed how you feel in the morning after binging on processed food? Food can have a direct impact on our mood. Eating too much sugar can lead to a crash shortly after making us feel tired or irritable, while drinking lots of caffeine can make us feel anxious and effect our sleep. Our daily food choices can significantly influence how our day goes.

Let's break down the macronutrients which include proteins, carbohydrates, and fats.

Protein

Protein is a necessary component in any diet. Protein is important when it comes to making enzymes, antibodies (which fight viruses), connective tissue, and even neurotransmitters. Neurotransmitters, like serotonin (made from tryptophan, an amino acid) are important in mood regulation and can help us feel calm and relaxed? Think of that happy feeling that comes after eating a big turkey dinner.

It's recommended that adults consume 0.36 grams of protein for every pound of body weight daily. For example: If you weigh 150 pounds, you would multiply 150 x 0.36 to calculate your daily protein need in grams. So, a 150-pound adult would need about 54 grams of protein daily.

If you are over 60, an increase in daily protein intake is recommended to account for muscle mass loss. For athletes, the recommended daily amount is doubled.

Healthier Protein Options

Choose This	Not That
Grass-Fed Beef	Grain-Fed Beef
Organic chicken	Regular factory-raised Chicken
Wild salmon	Farmed salmon
Organic, free-range eggs	Egg substitutes and/or regular eggs

Carbohydrates

There are simple carbohydrates and complex carbohydrates. Certain types of dietary fiber are also considered carbohydrates. Carbohydrates vary in their effects on blood sugar levels. The glycemic index is a way to quantify how carbohydrates impact blood glucose levels after consumption. For example: baked potatoes, jelly beans, or white bread are rapidly digested and will cause a rapid increase in glucose levels. This subsequently results in a spike in blood insulin levels which has also been shown to increase the risk for developing type 2 diabetes and cardiovascular disease. Oatmeal, apples, or broccoli are absorbed more slowly so the glucose levels rise more slowly while they are digested preventing a spike in insulin. As you can see, it's important to consider picking foods with a lower glycemic index. This helps your body maintain steady blood glucose levels which keeps you healthier!

Healthier Carbohydrate Options

Choose This	Instead of This
Sweet potato	Regular potato
Broccoli or Cauliflower rice	Rice
Black bean brownie	Regular brownie (with wheat flour)
Quinoa	Pasta

Fats

Fats are also important for our bodies. Besides helping with our basic bodily functions, fats are a key component of cell membranes and are precursors to biochemical mediators and hormone production. Dietary fats are classified based on the number of carbon-carbon bonds present in the fatty acids.

Saturated fats, such as butter or coconut oil, are solid at room temperature. Polyunsaturated fats include omega-3 and omega-6 fatty acids. Both are important for supporting proper, healthy brain and heart function. Keep in mind we need to have a proper ratio of omega-3 to omega-6.

Examples of oils high in omega-6 are sunflower oil, corn oil, and soybean oil. These should not be used for high-temperature cooking because they can form toxic lipid peroxides (basically, damaged lipid molecules) which can result in protein and DNA damage within cells. Unfortunately, however, soybean oil is frequently used in restaurants for frying foods. Omega-3 fatty acids have cardio-protective and anti-inflammatory effects. Having too much omega-6 fatty acids can throw off the balance in the body. We want a healthy ratio of omega-3 to omega-6 acids, or chronic inflammation can occur. Extra virgin olive oil is an example of a healthy oil to cook with that is also high in omega-3 fatty acids. Avocado oil, another monosaturated fat, can also be used to cook with.

We should completely avoid trans fatty acids that contain

artificial ingredients (e.g., margarine). Trans fats have been linked to coronary artery disease (heart disease), an increase in total cholesterol, and lowering of HDL cholesterol (the good cholesterol).

Healthier Fat Options

Choose This	Not That
Olive oil	Canola Oil
Avocado Oil	Sunflower or Soy oil
Almond butter	Cream Cheese
Grass-fed butter (higher in gut-healthy butyric acid)	Butter (lower in omega-3 and vitamin K2)

By the Numbers

Now that we have a basic understanding of macronutrients, (Protein, Carbs, Fat) let's take a quick look at the caloric numbers, starting with the basics.

What's a calorie, anyway? In foods, a calorie is a unit of measurement. A calorie tells us the amount of energy required to raise 1 gram of water by 1 degree Celsius. We need calories to burn so we can move and function. Different types of foods have different amounts of calories.

PROTEIN: 4 calories of energy per gram

CARBS: 4 calories of energy per gram

FAT: 9 calories of energy per gram

TYPES OF DIETS

L et's break down some of the more popular diets.

Like we mentioned before, the focus is more on a lifestyle change than a diet. A diet often leads to restriction and later bingeing, which can take a significant toll on our motivation. It is far more important to incorporate a lifestyle change that you are capable of maintaining and will lead to a better quality of life. Our goal is to help you eat your way to more energy and better health.

Mediterranean Diet

This popular diet is well researched and known for its protective effects against cardiovascular disease, role in boosting cognitive health (your brain's ability to think), and cancer prevention. The many benefits of this diet most likely stem from the high amount of healthy fats, including olive oil (a healthy omega-3 fat). Let's break it down!

Vegetables: 4 or more servings each day

Fruits: 3 or more servings each day

Grains : 4 or more servings each day

Fats/Oils: Olive Oil - 4 tablespoons or more each day

Nuts/Seeds: 3 or more servings each week

Beans/Legumes: 3 or more servings each week

Fish and Seafood: 2-3 servings each week

Herbs and Spices: use daily

Yogurt/Cheese/Egg Poultry: daily to weekly

Alcohol/Wine: Men — 1-2 glasses each day; Women - 1 glass each day

Here's an example of what a daily menu might look like if you were practicing the Mediterranean Diet:

Breakfast: steel-cut oats with blueberries and walnuts

Snack: banana or apple

Lunch: mixed greens, chickpeas, onions, carrots, olives, cucumbers, feta cheese, organic sprouted bread, salad dressing (olive oil & balsamic vinegar)

Dinner: salmon, brown rice, roasted broccoli in olive oil

Snack: almonds

Beverages: water, sparkling water, green tea, one glass of red wine

Atkins Diet

Atkins is a low-carbohydrate diet. With suggestions like bacon for breakfast and pork rinds for a snack, it's easy to see why this diet garnered a lot of popularity. The Atkins Diet, introduced by cardiologist Robert Atkins, MD, emphasizes animal foods, eggs, cheese, and low-carbohydrate vegetables. It does not restrict caloric intake. There are two things to consider with the Atkins Diet. The low carb intake can significantly help with quicker weight loss. However, the long-term safety remains questionable with this diet lifestyle. While it might not do damage to our heart or kidneys in the short-term, there is potential for harm in the long run.

Here's an example of what a daily menu might look like eating the Atkins Diet:

Breakfast: bacon and eggs

Snack: carrots or celery with Ranch salad dressing

Lunch: flank steak and broccoli cooked in olive oil

Snack: low carb snack bar

Dinner: hamburger (no bun) with pepper-jack cheese, avocado, lettuce, and sliced tomato

Beverages: water, tea, no-calorie drinks

Paleo Diet

Eating like a caveman? That's the gist of the Paleo Diet. Early humans were primarily hunters and gatherers. They didn't regularly harvest grains and they weren't baking bread. If we're following this diet, food choices are guided by the principle that if our Paleolithic ancestors didn't eat it, we shouldn't either. Research on the Paleo Diet has shown improvement in weight loss, blood pressure, and triglycerides (elevated triglycerides have been shown to increase risk of stroke, heart attack, and heart disease).[ii] This diet places an emphasis on foods that can be hunted (fish and meat) or gathered (tree nuts, eggs, vegetables, fruits, berries). Raw honey, coconut sugar, olive oil, ghee, and coconut oil are all acceptable. Dairy, grains, sugar, legumes, rice, white potatoes, and processed oils are all strictly avoided.

The daily menu while practicing the Paleo Diet might include:

Breakfast: spinach omelet cooked in coconut oil, fresh raspberries

Snack: apple with almond butter

Lunch: chicken salad with avocado and onions, fresh blueberries

Dinner: steak, cauliflower rice with coconut aminos,

roasted sweet potato

Snack: dates with walnuts

Beverages: water, herbal tea, coffee

Vegetarian Diet

Let's make one key distinction: Vegan vs. Vegetarian. What's the difference?

Vegan: Consumes no animal products. Period.

Vegetarian: Does not eat animals, but may eat products that come from animals (eggs, dairy, honey)

The Vegetarian Diet is fairly self-explanatory. Load up on plenty of fruits, vegetables, legumes, and healthy grains. However, keep in mind, that while vegetarians have a lower incidence of cardiovascular disease, hypertension, kidney stones, and diabetes (compared to most omnivores), they may be low in micronutrients. If you follow a Vegetarian Diet, some supplementation may be necessary to ensure you're getting sufficient amounts of vitamin B12, iron, vitamin D, zinc, iodine, riboflavin, calcium, and selenium.[iii]

Along with a bevy of vegetables, here are some popular food choices for the Vegetarian Diet:

- quinoa and pumpkin seeds

- all-natural nut butter on whole-grain bread

- rice and beans

- soybeans with soba noodles

- Ezekiel bread with almond butter

- brown rice with mushrooms and herbs

Low-FODMAPs Diet

"FODMAPs" is an acronym for Fermentable Oligosaccharides, Disaccharides, Monosaccharides, And Polyols. Quite a mouthful. I know what you may be thinking. In plain English, please.

At its most basic, the Low FODMAP[iv] Diet cuts out certain carbohydrates that can cause or trigger irritable bowel syndrome (IBS). This diet is low in FODMAPs which include fructose, lactose, sorbitol, fructans (fructooligosaccharides, inulin), and galactans (also called galactooligosaccharides; e.g., raffinose). It's been shown to help people like my patient Amy, whom I discussed earlier, and can improve the symptoms of irritable bowel syndrome, bloating, or abdominal pain.

Here's an example of eating the Low-FODMAP diet:

<u>Breakfast</u>: steel-cut oats, almond milk, strawberries

Snack: pumpkin seeds and cucumber slices

Lunch: salmon, quinoa, spinach, olive oil

Dinner: grilled chicken with spaghetti squash and tomato sauce

Snack: 1-piece dairy-free >70% dark chocolate

AIP Diet

The autoimmune protocol diet (AIP) is a strict diet used to help decrease inflammation in the body and improve gut health. You are allowed to eat vegetables except for night-shades (e.g., potatoes, tomatoes, peppers, eggplant), fruits, protein, and healthy fats. However, on the AIP diet, you strictly avoid grains, dairy, soy, nuts, seeds, legumes, night-shades, eggs, additives, and artificial sugars.

That's quite a list! But on the bright side, studies have shown the AIP Diet improves symptoms in patients suffering from irritable bowel syndrome (IBS)[v] and decreases inflammatory markers.[vi]

An example of eating the AIP Diet:

Breakfast: turkey sausage with blueberries

Snack: apples and cucumber slices

Lunch: salmon salad with olive oil dressing

Dinner: Chicken Marsala (use tapioca starch)

Snack: bone broth with chicken, carrots, celery, and onions

Ketogenic Diet

Often called Keto, the Ketogenic Diet was originally used to help patients with seizure disorders. Now, the Keto Diet is very popular for effective weight loss. Like Atkins, Keto is higher in fats and protein, and allows low amounts of carbs. There are other benefits to this diet. The Ketogenic Diet promotes a non-atherogenic lipid profile, lowers blood pressure, and improves glucose and insulin levels.[vii] What this means is, cholesterol is going to be less likely to form plaques, which can lead to heart disease and heart attacks. This diet also has anti-neoplastic (anti-cancer) benefits. It has been shown not to alter kidney or liver function or produce metabolic acidosis, meaning that people on this diet will have lab work still in a normal range if the diet is followed correctly. Ketosis has possible neurological benefits in the central nervous system, including decreasing inflammation, while slowing osteoporosis. If that's not enough, the Keto Diet may even increase performance in aerobic sports like swimming, running, and Zumba.

Here's an example of a daily menu eating the Ketogenic

Diet:

Breakfast: eggs cooked in coconut oil with bacon

Snack: grass-fed beef stick

Lunch: grilled salmon on romaine lettuce with avocado oil, Ranch dressing

Dinner: grass-fed steak, side of broccoli cooked in butter

Snack: hardboiled egg

Beverages: water, tea, butter coffee

Whole 30 Diet

The Whole-30 Diet is an elimination-style eating plan that eliminates common trigger foods. Soy, dairy, grains, alcohol, legumes, and added sugars are strictly removed from the diet. After 30 days, when the body is at a baseline, these foods are slowly introduced back into the diet, one at a time. By slowly re-introducing foods, you can take note of any particular trigger foods that cause allergic, inflammatory, or negative responses in your body.

Here's an example of what a menu looks like on the Whole-30 Diet:

Breakfast: smoked salmon and poached eggs

Snack: mixed nuts and salami

<u>Lunch</u>: taco lettuce wraps with plantain chips and salsa

<u>Dinner</u>: zucchini noodles with avocado pesto and shrimp

<u>Snack</u>: dates and walnuts (or a fruit and nut bar such as Larabar™)

<u>Beverages</u>: purified water

Intermittent & Modified Fasting

Fasting is typically seen as a hypo-caloric diet. Hypo-caloric is just a technical way of saying there's a reduction in daily food or calories. Dietary restriction means purposely not eating at certain times of the day or evening. There are different strategies of when to eat and when to fast. How long should the fasting window be?

In short, fasting means not eating any food. Consuming water, black coffee, and tea may be allowed, as long as they do not contain calories. But keep in mind, some religious fasting does not allow for the consumption of anything during the fasting period.

Traditional Fasting has been part of religious ceremonies for thousands of years. Traditional fasting restricts eating between certain periods of the day. Therefore, the number of calories is often less because the number of hours to consume meals is reduced.

Clinical Fasting is fasting typically done under medical supervision with a low daily caloric intake (200–900 kcal nutritional intake/day) for periods of seven to 21 days. Done under clinical supervision, this fast has been shown to help with medical issues such as depression and rheumatoid arthritis.[viii]

Intermittent Fasting can be defined as time-restricted eating. This type of fasting is focused on reducing the window of time for eating and increasing the window of time for fasting within a 24-hour period. An example of this would be waiting to eat a first meal until noon. The benefits and results of intermittent fasting may vary depending on the number and timing of meals. Additionally, portioning your entire intake into two meals without changing your total energy consumption (meaning activity for the day) may have beneficial effects on the inflammatory markers associated with metabolic syndrome.[ix] Metabolic syndrome is defined as high blood sugar, high blood pressure, abnormal cholesterol levels, and excess body fat around the waist.

Intermittent fasting and reducing the amount of time engaged in food consumption (time-restricted eating) appears to have some of the same results as traditional fasting. This includes reducing oxidative stress (the ability of our biological system to detoxify reactive oxygen species which can harm our cells) and decreasing pro-inflammatory cytokines which if chronically elevated result in inflammation that can cause damage to our cells and tissues[x].

There are lots of benefits to an intermittent fast. It could be as simple as having an earlier dinner and skipping breakfast the next day. Time-restricted and intermittent fasting are commonly practiced by using an "eating window." In a 24-hour day, you fast for 16 consecutive hours and then eat during the next eight hours. That would be a 16:8 window, 16 off, eight on. Another common practice is an 18:6 window. 18 hours fasting, six hours eating. More extreme examples are 20:4 or even 22:2. But whatever window you choose, it's recommended to have at least 12 hours of fasting overnight to allow the gut to rest and for autophagy (recycling and removal of old cell material), to take place. The process of autophagy is crucial for a healthy body. While it might sound challenging, you may find that intermittent fasting is easier than you think and a habit that you can build over time.

Here's an example of a 16:8 fast. Your eating window is noon-8pm:

Breakfast: skip; drink water, organic tea, organic black coffee

<u>Lunch</u>: eat something sensible (such as an omelet, smoothie, or salmon salad) starting at noon

<u>Snack</u>: whatever you'd like, as needed (such as almonds or a grass-fed beef stick)

<u>Dinner</u>: something sensible, but nothing after 8p

WHICH DIET IS RIGHT FOR ME?

If you are looking to try one of these diets, contact your physician and a dietician before you make any major lifestyle changes. Your local library is also a great resource. Internet searches for more information about these specific diets may be helpful. There are countless books and reputable magazines that can offer more detailed information on each of these diets. You can also find a host of tasty menu ideas, meal plans, and delicious recipes online and in print.

Do keep this in mind: whichever diet you try, you will want to stick with it for at least one month to receive the benefits. Remember, make it a lifestyle. This isn't a fad. It's a choice for you and your family to live healthier and more active lives.

The Usual Suspects

Do you sometimes feel terrible after eating out? Do you find yourself wanting to take a power nap after that drive-thru lunch? Ask yourself, what are you putting into your body? If it's processed food, toxins, and refined sugars, there's a reason your body feels that crash. Garbage in.

Garbage out.

What should you avoid? What should go into your shopping cart and what should stay on the shelf? Let's answer these questions.

We've already identified foods that can be beneficial to our health and foods that are not. But what exactly makes some food toxic for us? After all, a calorie is just a calorie.

Unfortunately, our body doesn't process all calories the same way. When our body is faced with chemicals it doesn't need, it will put significant energy into detoxing and purging instead of focusing on keeping the body healthy. This can mean decreased energy, decreased immune function, and increased stress on the body. Some foods can cause us to pack on pounds and become overweight which can lead to a host of additional health risks.

The following are some of the usual suspects in greater detail. If you see these ingredients on the label, don't even think about it. Put it back on the shelf.

Artificial Dyes

Ever wonder why your children acted out after a Halloween party? Why they were acting crazy at that birthday party? Why their sleep was off? Well, food dyes could be to blame. Artificial food dyes are chemicals not found in natural food sources. We are naturally attracted to bright colors. We reach for brightly colored packages over plain colored ones. The same principle applies to what we put in our mouth. However, when it comes to food dyes, it comes at a price.

So which dyes have been shown to cause negative outcomes?

Meet public enemy number one: **Yellow No. 5**

This bad boy is loaded into candy, breakfast cereals, sodas, and much more. It gives a yellow color but can also be used in green items. Studies show this food dye, also called tartrazine, when combined with sodium benzoate (a common food preservative), can cause irritability, restlessness, and sleep disturbances in children.[xi] Is your child eating this each morning in their breakfast cereal? What about that popsicle or that fruit-flavored drink? Read that label again. It might be time to swap out those Fruit Loops so your child can have a better day at school.

Red dye 40.

Red dye 40 is found in a variety of foods from Doritos™ and M&Ms™, to salad dressing. This additive is proven to increase hyperactivity in children.[xii]

Ask any teacher after a classroom birthday party with red icing cupcakes; it's worse than just a sugar high. And it's only getting worse. The consumption of artificial food coloring has quadrupled in the past fifty years.[xiii]

These chemicals affect the brain and should be avoided if possible. In the words of the Greek philosopher, Paracelsus, "The dose makes the poison."

So, what should we do? First, check the label on the products you consume. Avoid additives altogether if you can. Look for natural colorings such as spirulina, beetroot, and turmeric. And consider this last nugget when making your food choices: When children with ADHD (attention-deficit/hyperactivity disorder) were put on an elimination diet removing preservatives and artificial colors, they showed improvement in their ADHD symptoms.[xiv]

Artificial Flavorings & Additives

It might not be your fault that you want to eat McDonald's™ all the time. And there's a good reason why. Once you pop that can of chips, you can't stop shoving them into your mouth. These foods are chemically engineered to trigger the reward center of our brains. Like an addictive drug, they make us crave more. The hidden culprit is food additives, just like red dye 40, which has been shown to increase ADHD symptoms in children. Even worse, some studies are suggesting food additives may play a causal role in the development of ADHD[xv].

So, what is a food additive? In short, it's something added to your food to enhance its taste, flavor, or appearance. Some examples are nitrites, nitrates, potassium bromate, BHT, propylparaben, and diacetyl. But one of the most dangerous forms of food additives is hiding in plain sight (and your pantry).

Sugar. Did you know sugar activates the same pleasure areas of your brain as cocaine? It's true. Sugar is highly pleasurable and equally addictive, and that might be part of the reason why it's everywhere. It's in your coffee, your ketchup, your soup, your bread, but it's even worse than that. Sugar has many names when added to foods. It hides under aliases like corn syrup, high fructose corn syrup, malt sugar, turbinado sugar, glucose, cane syrup, fructose, mannose, sugar beet, and more.

Why is sugar so bad?

First, sugar is very inflammatory. Chronic inflammation has been shown to cause cellular and tissue damage which can lead to the development of diseases (e.g., heart disease, bowel diseases, arthritis) or even cancer. Americans consume 16.1% of their total calories from added sugars, and consumption is growing.[xvi] Because sugar is addictive and we crave it, we have a hard time cutting it out. Our craving for sugar leads us to binge-eat high sugar foods[xvii].

On the tongue, sugar is highly palatable. It's an instant reward, both in taste and providing an immediate energy boost. However, consuming excessive sugar triggers neuro-adaptations in the reward system that decouples eating behavior from caloric needs. In other words, because sugar targets the part of the brain that causes pleasure, you eat way more of it than you need (e.g., that pint of Ben & Jerry's™ ice cream).

The science behind overeating and sugar is alarming. There is a clear link between regularly eating high-sugar foods and compulsive overeating. Excessive sugar intake is, in turn, associated with adverse health conditions including obesity, high blood pressure, diabetes, bad choles-terol, and heart disease.[xviii]

In a study of rats eating sugar, researchers concluded sugar was more addictive than cocaine.[xix] The rats' brains were more rewarded when regularly given sugar than when regularly given cocaine. The rats consistently chose the sweet substance over highly addictive cocaine[xx].

Most studies are concerned with added sugar and addi-tives, like sucrose and fructose. These additives were not in our ancestors' diets, but are now found in most processed foods. The more sugars and additives we eat, the more we crave. We are constantly stuck in that hamster wheel, chasing after the next sugar high. When we consider the evidence linking high sugar consumption to obesity, metabolic syndrome, and the development of diabetes, this is a catastrophic feedback loop.

But it gets worse. Say hello to **high fructose corn syrup (HFCS).**

If sugar is a wave, high fructose corn syrup is a tsunami. This additive can crash your health and that of your children. It's cheap. It's manufactured. It's in everything.

HFCS is linked to obesity and an increased risk of colorectal cancer[xxi]. Another concern is high fructose corn syrup's involvement in the development of nonalcoholic fatty liver disease (NASH)[xxii]. Beverages containing high fructose corn syrup, such as soda, have been linked to weight gain and an increased risk of obesity—simply by drinking soda for six months[xxiii]. One study showed the visceral fat, the "spare tire" of fat around your waist, was the area affected the most. This fat is the most harmful type of body fat and is linked to health issues such as heart disease and diabetes. Consuming food or drinks with HFCS can also increase inflammation in the body and increase the risk for gout, a painful joint disease.[xxiv]

Fructose has also been noted to increase food-seeking

behavior and increase fat production and fat storage.[xxv] Another concern is the link between high fructose corn syrup and fatty liver disease. Nonalcoholic liver disease (liver disease not caused by drinking alcohol) can lead to liver cirrhosis, also known as liver failure. High fructose corn syrup is bad news, do not take it lightly. It's best to stay away from this addictive food additive.

PROCESSED FOODS & HIGH GLYCEMIC INDEX

Here's the problem with quick, cheap, processed foods. They're packed with additives, sugars, and preservatives. After we eat them, they often leave us hungry again, sometimes within an hour. Foods with a high glycemic index will raise your blood sugar quickly (which also raises your insulin) and lead to a crash in energy levels. If you pick a low glycemic index food (foods with more fat and fiber), you will feel fuller longer and not experience that crash.

Not only does eating processed foods with a high glycemic index make you feel bad, it can also cause drastic fluctuations in your blood glucose levels. This can eventually lead to the development of diabetes. This is why it's essential to choose foods with a lower glycemic index. These food choices have more fiber in them.

When offered a choice, go for fresh foods over dried foods. Fresh fruits, for example, contain more fiber and usually have a lower glycemic index than dried foods. Think of eating a handful of grapes versus a handful of raisins. As

I'm sure you've noticed, when you're hungry, you eat fewer grapes to feel full than if you're snacking on raisins. The same goes for juices. Think about how many oranges you need to eat to feel satisfied versus how many go into one glass of orange juice?

Low Glycemic Index Foods (Green = Go)

Broccoli, Celery, Peas

Apple, Pear, Grapes

Carrots, Black beans

Medium Glycemic Index Foods (Yellow = Caution)

Corn, Banana

Sweet potato, White rice

Raisins, Table sugar

High Glycemic Index Foods (Red = Stop)

White bread, Potatoes

French fries, Doughnuts

Jelly beans, Dates

Artificial Sweeteners

We know sugar is bad for us, so maybe grabbing a diet soda would seem like the next best option. Not so fast!

Artificial sweeteners are also bad news. Most are highly processed. Stay away from sucralose, aspartame, and Splenda. Not only are they riddled with chemicals, but they also might make you fat! Yes, you read that right.

Researchers in one study looked at the link between artificial sweeteners and obesity. What they found was artificial sweeteners appear to change the host gut microbiome, alter glucose homeostasis within the body, lead to a decreased sense of being full, and were associated with increased caloric intake and weight gain.[xxvi] It seems counterintuitive, but trying to save calories by consuming fake sugar can actually cause more damage.

Caffeine & Alcohol

Like most things in life, moderation is a wise choice when it comes to caffeine and alcohol use. It's also a good idea to use caution. These drugs have different effects on the body. Caffeine is a stimulant, while alcohol is a depressant. Caffeine is an addictive food and can increase anxiety in some users. Obviously, if it's consumed later in the day it can interfere with sleep. If you are going to have your coffee in the morning, consider swapping it out for something healthier. Give green tea a try, but try to limit yourself to just one cup.

Alcohol has its own side effects to consider. Excessive alcohol intake contributes to a number of health concerns including hepatitis, cirrhosis, cardiomyopathy, depression, dementia, and nutritional deficiencies. However, it is widely believed that moderate alcohol consumption (1 drink per day for women, 2 drinks per day for men) isn't harmful for most people. In fact, some studies show a small drink may reduce the risk of developing cardiovascular disease. Also known as "The French Paradox", there is some research to suggest that one glass of wine, which contains antioxidants, might be beneficial.[xxvii] Nevertheless, the purported cardio-protective effect of alcohol is based primarily on observational studies and is still open to debate. The message is simple: When it comes to consuming addictive substances like caffeine and alcohol, caution is recommended.

Pesticides & Herbicides

This one is pretty straightforward. If an insect doesn't want to eat the vegetation because it's been sprayed with a poison, you probably shouldn't ingest it. The serious and grave health risks of pesticides and herbicides have been widely described. You've probably seen a commercial or two about cancer lawsuits involving weed killers. Our concern is how can we avoid these poisons on our food? What can you do to avoid pesticides in our food and while grocery shopping?

For starters, go to the Environmental Working Group, or EWG.org website and download the shopping list for fruits and vegetables. They've trademarked them as the *Clean 15* and the *Dirty 12*. Write them down (they change seasonally) and pick up the clean ones when you go grocery shopping. It's an easy fix. If the recommended foods are not available where you shop, there are still steps you can take to mitigate exposure to pesticides.

Obviously, buying organic helps. Organic producers have stricter guidelines to follow in the production of their foods. However, being certified organic does not mean the food is chemical and pesticide-free at harvest. When you get your produce home, make sure you wash it off. A vinegar soak is ideal.

High Dietary Salt Intake

Sodium, by itself, can be deadly. Chloride, on its own, is lethal. When you chemically combine them, you get sodium chloride—table salt—an essential mineral in a healthy diet.

Such is the magic of chemistry. A high intake of salt is associated with an increased risk of obesity and hypertension. Those factors can lead to an increased risk of stroke and heart attack.[xxviii]

The World Health Organization (WHO) recommends salt consumption levels of less than five grams each day, but it has been estimated that the current intake of salt in most countries of the world is 9-12 grams daily.

Why is this a problem?

It's estimated that 50-60% of people with hypertension are salt-sensitized. There is research suggesting that the elderly and overweight populations gain the most benefit by decreasing their salt intake. Reduce your salt and you reduce the risk for cardiovascular disease.[xxix] One diet, the Dietary Approaches to Stop Hypertension (DASH), has been helpful for people who are at risk for cardiovascular disease. The DASH diet recommends foods lower in sodium and foods rich in potassium, magnesium, and calcium. These nutrients also aid in lowering blood pressure. On this diet, you consume vegetables, fruits, whole grains, fish, poultry, and nuts. And in moderation, you can add meats, red wine, and even some sweets.

Salt is necessary in our diet and is a great way to add flavor to vegetables. However, it's the hidden sodium, the salt added to processed foods, that is harmful to our long-term health. If you're cooking your own food, season lightly. If you're eating processed food, read the labels carefully. How many grams of salt are hiding in there?

Helpful Hint:

A pinch of salt contains about 400 mg of sodium!

Soybean & Canola Oils

If you read a bottle of vegetable oil, it will often claim that it's great for making salad dressing. Guess what? These oils aren't good for you. In fact, soybean oil has been linked to obesity and diabetes.

A recent study found that feeding mice soybean oil had profound effects on the hypothalamus, the part of the brain that regulates metabolism and hunger, among many other functions.[xxx] The soybean-fed mice developed health issues including obesity, diabetes, insulin resistance, and fatty liver disease. Scientists have also linked soybean oil to neurological conditions like autism, depression, anxiety, and even Alzheimer's disease. Levels of oxytocin, produced in the hypothalamus and known as the "love hormone," decreased in soybean oil-fed mice.

Think about it. You eat a bunch of fries cooked in GMO (genetically modified organism) soybean oil from a fast food place. Your hypothalamus goes haywire, the feel-good oxytocin hormone decreases, you feel sad, and to manage these feelings, you eat more. Then what? You start feeling terrible. You get sluggish and gain a bunch of weight, but you're sitting there depressed, ordering more fried food to feel better. Now you're depressed and overweight, have insulin resistance and fatty liver disease. While this is a simplistic analysis of how some foods can impact us, there is some truth to it. Consider how frequently antidepressants, such as Zoloft (an antidepressant classified as a Selective Serotonin Reuptake Inhibitor, SSRI) are prescribed. Could it be that our food might be impacting us in ways we don't realize? Do yourself—and your liver—a favor; pass on foods cooked in soybean oil.

What about canola oil?

Like other vegetable oils, canola oil is highly processed. It goes through an extensive refining process to make it an oil. This process involves chemicals to bleach the rapeseed first, and then more chemicals for degumming. The solvent manufacturers typically use hexane. In the final steps of the refinement process, the oil is deodorized, which involves even more chemicals. Simply put, the entire process to make canola oil involves the addition of a variety of chemicals.

Oils that are cold-pressed are better, but these are harder to find and more expensive. Canola and soybean oil are cheap to make. That's why you see them in many cheap, convenient food products, which are often highly processed foods. Cold-pressed oils are made by the physical pressing of the products instead of using heat and chemicals. A few examples of cold-pressed oils include avocado oil and olive oil. The important point to remember is to avoid highly processed and chemical-filled oils and foods. Your body will thank you.

STRATEGIES FOR GROCERY SHOPPING

L et's keep this simple, too. Consider these two
principles when you shop at the grocery store:

Buy food.

Don't buy products.

To accomplish this, stay on the perimeter of the grocery
store. This is where you'll find the healthier foods, produce,
fruits, meats, and fish. It's the inner aisles where you'll get
into trouble. The inside aisles of most grocery stores are
filled with a maze of processed food, including chips,
cereals, canned goods loaded with salt, or frozen meals full
of preservatives. Stay out of the middle. Be an outsider!

Most grocery stores now have organic options next to the
"regular" items. Choose organic when you can. There will
be fewer pesticides and unnecessary ingredients. If you *have*
to buy processed foods, read the labels. Avoid food dyes,
artificial flavors, bad oils, and hidden sugars. Most food
products that come in a package will be loaded with junk.

Beware of salad dressings. When you read the label, you'll
find that many of them contain additives. Keep an eye out

for high fructose corn syrup, food dyes, bad oils, and sodium. If you're shopping with your family, ask them to help out. Have them read the labels with you; for kids, make it a game. Look for hidden oils, hidden artificial food coloring, or hidden sugar. Now that you're looking for them, you will be amazed at how many of those products are in foods.

Limit buying snacks like potato chips, soda, sweets, and fruit snacks. They're packed full of junk. If it's in the house, you or someone in your family will be tempted to eat it. Instead, save those items for special occasions.

Focus on veggies and fresh fruit, and your body will thank you. Sometimes frozen vegetables are a great option. Since they are picked fresh and then quickly frozen, they can still have great flavor even if they are out of season. Remember, when you begin shopping for healthy foods it may take you longer since you're reading the labels. However, the more you do it, the easier it will become.

Another great way to shop for produce is to utilize your local farmers' market. By shopping for farm-to-table food, you are supporting your local economy. You can find all the vegetables you need there, fresh and in season. Plus, most markets carry other local items like berries, eggs, meat, and honey. Check to see when and where your farmers' market occurs and make it a habit to visit.

Let's recap. Use these strategies at the grocery store to make stronger food choices:

- Stay on the perimeter

- Read the labels

- Load up on veggies

- Buy food, not products

Food as Medicine

Clark came to me after being diagnosed with colon cancer. He was frustrated with his energy levels and wanted to optimize his health while going through cancer treatments. Unfortunately, his cancer doctors were not giving him sound advice on nutrition. When he came to me, he was following their instructions and still eating canned and processed foods. I spoke with him about how nutrition is key for health and to think of food as medicine. What we put into our bodies has the potential to either heal disease or create disease. Everything we put in our mouths is going to either help fight cancer or promote cancer. Each bite will either reduce inflammation or produce it.

After our talk, Clark changed his diet. He eliminated the highly processed foods. He invested in a juicer. Most importantly, he paid more attention to how the foods he ate made him feel. To round things off, we also added supplements to support his digestion. He worked hard at changing his diet and increasing anti-inflammatory foods. And the work paid off. By making better food choices, Clark felt better and had more energy.

When he arrived for his follow up appointment, I was floored. He looked amazing and his cancer had not progressed. What a difference the fuel we put in our body makes. By focusing on simple nutritional habits, Clark was feeling so much better. Good, healthy food is the glue that holds a healthy body together.

Let's Get Cooking

If cooking was easy, everybody would save money and do it. The truth is, it can take a lot of work to cook your own meals. With our busy schedules, home cooking can be overwhelming. However, it can also be rewarding and a lot of fun.

To make healthy meals at home, you need a stovetop, oven, pans, and a few other basic cooking utensils and goods. Olive oil is a great fat. You can use it to sauté, roast, and bake. Olive oil is also packed with heart-healthy omega-3 fatty acids.

Crockpots are a great tool for cooking at home and for

making nutrient-dense chili at home. Beans are an excellent source of protein and fiber. Tomatoes are packed with phytonutrients such as lycopene. Add in grass-fed meat for protein, and onions for Vitamin C and folate. Toss all the ingredients into the crock pot in the morning and it's done for dinnertime. Another great use for the crockpot is shredded chicken. Place the chicken breast in the crockpot in the morning, and you'll have shredded chicken when you return home from work. It's great on salads, in casseroles, and more. Chicken thighs which contain more fat, also cook well in the crockpot.

Instapots are also great kitchen tools for the reluctant chef. Cooking vegetables in the Instapot is one of the best ways to cook vegetables since more nutrients are retained. Instapots can also steam rice, cook quinoa, meat, chicken, and much more. You can even make homemade soup stocks and bone broths in it.

Don't be afraid to get in the kitchen and give home cooking a try. It's easier than you think. Heat up your veggies until they are tender and season them lightly. Toss some greens with a few of your favorite chopped vegetables and herbs and drizzle with some olive oil and dash of vinegar. That's all there is to it. You're on your way.

RECIPE IDEAS

Here are a few recipes to get you started. For more ideas and international flavors, browse the internet, visit a book store, or peruse your local library. There are millions of recipes at your fingertips.

<u>Salad Dressing</u>

½ cup extra virgin olive oil

¼ cup apple cider vinegar

½ cup local honey

1 tsp dried basil

¼ tsp sea salt

- Mix together and serve on a salad.

<u>GF (gluten-free)/DF (dairy-free) Banana Bread</u>

(makes two loaves)

2 cups gluten-free flour blend (or almond flour + 1/2 tsp xanthan gum)

1 tsp baking soda

½ tsp salt

6 overripe bananas, mashed

2 eggs

1 ½ cups organic sugar

½ cup organic maple syrup

½ cup melted coconut oil

½ cup dairy-free chocolate chips

(I added a touch of ground flaxseed and oatmeal to boost my milk production because I am breastfeeding, but these are healthy for everyone!)

- Mash the bananas first, add the "wet" ingredients, then add the dry ingredients. Mix and pour batter into two loaf pans.

- Bake at 350 degrees for 45 - 60 minutes (until a toothpick comes out clean).

Baking with small kids means keeping recipes simple and in one bowl. It still turns out yummy!

Homemade Gummies

1 cup 100% organic fruit juice

2-3 tbsp honey

6 tbsp gelatin

- Mix fruit juice, honey, and gelatin in a pan on the stove and warm until all the gelatin is dissolved.

- Use medicine droppers to transfer to molds, or pour into molds.

- Place in the fridge until solid.

- Push out of the molds and refrigerate what you don't use.

Tips: Add the gelatin slowly while mixing so it won't clump together. For your beverage, pick a fruit juice with no added sugar.

Cucumber Cilantro Salad

2 cucumbers peeled and sliced

1 chopped onion

Fresh cilantro (as you prefer)

Lime juice (from one lime)

2 tsp apple cider vinegar

4 tsp extra virgin olive oil

$\frac{1}{2}$ tsp garlic powder

Pinch of Celtic salt

- Mix together and serve.

This recipe is refreshing for the summer and you can even put it in a glass mason jar and pack it for lunch.

"Iron Cookies" (Molasses cookies which are high in iron)

½ cup organic brown sugar

½ cup coconut oil (melted)

2 free-range, organic eggs

¼ cup blackstrap molasses

1 tsp ginger

1 tsp cinnamon

1 tsp non-aluminum baking soda

1 ½ cup GF flour blend

- Place in the refrigerator for one hour.

- Take them out and roll into balls.

- Roll each in sugar and flatten on baking sheet.

- Bake at 350 degrees for 10 minutes.

Chickpea Chocolate Chip Cookie Dough

1 can chickpeas (drained and rinsed well)

1 tsp vanilla extract

⅓ cup nut butter (almond, cashew, or peanut butter)

¼ cup brown sugar (may substitute with honey, maple syrup, or coconut sugar)

2 tsp ground flaxseed or oatmeal

(optional 1-3 tbsp almond milk if you need a smoother consistency)

- Add all the ingredients (except for the chocolate chips) to a food processor and blend until smooth consistency.

- Mix in the chocolate chips. (Enjoy Life™ mini chips are my favorite!).

- Store in the fridge and share (or don't share) with the family.

Black Bean Brownies

2 cans black beans, rinsed well

¼ cup oatmeal

½ cup natural sugar (I used a mix of maple syrup and

honey)

2 eggs

½ cup raw cacao powder

¼ cup coconut oil, melted

1 tsp non-aluminum baking powder

- Blend all ingredients in a food processor until smooth.

- Grease an 8" x 8" baking pan with coconut oil or line with parchment paper.

- Bake at 350 degrees for 30 - 35 minutes.

- Top with chocolate chips.

Share with friends and don't tell them the secret ingredient.

Golden Milk

2 cups unsweetened coconut milk

2 tsp raw honey

½ tsp cinnamon

1 tsp turmeric

- Stir while bringing to a low boil on the stove.

- Let cool to drinking temperature and enjoy.

Play around with this recipe and make it your own! Maple syrup can be used instead of honey or substitute the coconut milk for almond.

Egg Roll in a Bowl

6-8 cups shredded cabbage

½ - 1 lb ground sausage

1 onion, diced

1 cup carrot, shredded

Optional ingredients:

¼ cup sprouts

½ cup green peas

1 egg, scrambled

Top with coconut aminos or GF soy sauce

- Cook sausage in a pan and set aside.

- Scramble egg and set aside.

- Sauté vegetables, stirring frequently, until cooked.

- Mix all ingredients together and serve with gluten-free soy sauce or coconut aminos.

Peanut Butter Pie

8 oz dairy-free cream cheese (the cleanest you can find)

½ tub of dairy-free whipped cream

½ cup peanut butter

¼ cup coconut sugar

¼ cup maple syrup

- Place all ingredients in a bowl and mix well.

- Place in a serving bowl and top with organic chocolate syrup and dairy-free chocolate chips.

You can use graham crackers to dip or pour mix in a gluten-free graham cracker crust.

If you pour in a pre-made, gluten-free graham cracker crust, refrigerate for 4 hours before serving!

Chicken Paprikash

2 lb organic chicken

1 onion

6 tbsp butter, ghee, or coconut oil

1 carton (32 oz) organic chicken stock or bone broth (bone broth can be made at home!)

8 oz dairy-free sour cream (or regular sour cream)

4 - 6 tbsp paprika

- Cut chicken breast into bite-size pieces, set aside.

- Place 4 tbsp butter or ghee into an oven-safe pan and sauté onions until soft.

- Add 2 tbsp more of butter or ghee and add chicken.

- Cook on both sides until brown.

- Add chicken stock, sour cream, and paprika.

- Mix well.

- Cook at 350 degrees for 45 minutes.

Serve with gluten-free pasta.

One Last Reminder on Diet...

Say yes!	No way!
Whole, unprocessed foods	Refined sugars, refined carbs
Grass-fed beef	Trans fat, fast food
Organic, free-range eggs and chicken	Factory eggs and chicken
Organic fruits and vegetables	Canned fruits and veggies with added sugar and salt
Herbs and spices to enhance flavors	Food additives and salt
Sparkling water and tea	Excessive caffeine and alcohol

Final Thoughts

I know this seems like a lot of information, but even the smallest of actions can have an incredible impact on your health. Start small, but be consistent. Make one positive change each day for your health. Try to introduce one healthy food a month and cut out one unhealthy food a month. Try a new recipe each week and eat out one less time a week.

Pause before you buy something from the grocery store. Start reading the labels while you shop for groceries. Think twice before you order food when eating out. If you are eating out, look at the nutritional information and make an informed choice. When in doubt, just pick a protein and a steamed vegetable as a side. If you are going to order a salad, ask for olive oil and vinegar (or bring your own dressing with you). Swap out soda for an unsweetened tea. Drink plenty of clean, filtered water daily.

Children can be challenging, but if they see you eating healthy, they will follow your example. Continue to give them new fruits and vegetables; they might even learn to like foods they wouldn't eat before. Roasting, steaming, and sautéing are all different ways to cook your vegetables. Mix it up. Healthy food doesn't have to be boring!

And remember, food is medicine. What you put in your mouth is either creating inflammation or protecting your body against it. Consider the type of fuel you're putting in your tank.

SLEEP

The following is an example of work-related sleep deprivation.

Tim was a workaholic. He spent most of his day focusing on the different aspects of his job and paying little attention to himself. The one thing which became obvious was how regularly Tim was exhausted. He began snapping at coworkers and became someone that others in his office wanted to avoid. When I saw Tim for exhaustion, he was convinced that something was physically wrong with him. He wondered if he had cancer or was anemic. He believed there had to be a medical explanation.

When I began questioning his lifestyle, he noted that, on average, he worked 12 to 14-hour days in the office. He would then go home and continue working on his computer or watch TV until he fell asleep, usually around 1 am. Sometimes, he drank caffeine and exercised around 8 pm in order to get a little more work in before bedtime. Many nights, he would have two bourbon on the rocks which he felt helped him sleep. On average, Tim slept about 4-5 hours a night. His philosophy was, "I can sleep when I am dead."

This, unfortunately, is a much more common scenario than we would like to believe. We spend approximately a third of our lives asleep. [xxxi] That's great news if you're waking up refreshed after a deep and soothing rest. Unfortunately, many of us are not practicing good sleep habits. As a result, we may suffer from chronic fatigue, health issues, and low performance in our daily lives. This is an all-too-common problem. Approximately 30% of adults have one or more symptoms of insomnia, [xxxii] while 20-30% of infants, toddlers, and preschoolers experience frequent nighttime awakenings or bedtime problems.[xxxiii]

The National Sleep Foundation 2014 Sleep Health Index™ found that 45% of American adults reported they had poor or insufficient sleep affecting their daily activities at least once a week.[xxxiv] Another study by the University of Pennsylvania Perelman School of Medicine found that 25% of Americans experience acute insomnia each year, but 75% recover without developing chronic insomnia.[xxxv] While the percent recovery from insomnia sounds promising, a 2007 study found that self-reported complaints of insomnia were associated with an increased risk of coronary artery disease, heart attack, or death.[xxxvi]

A persistent lack of sleep can quite literally be killing you. In fact, sleep deprivation has been shown to weaken the immune system, decrease sex drive, increase the risk of diabetes and stroke, worsen mood, diminish the ability to focus, and decrease cognitive performance.[xxxvii]

If that's not enough to encourage you to take your sleep seriously, sleep researchers have also found that insomnia often presents in conjunction with an array of psychiatric diseases: depression, anxiety, PTSD, and others.[xxxviii] A lack of sleep puts you at risk for other long-term health risks, such as stroke and cardiovascular disease.[xxxix] Sleep loss has even been associated with age-specific increased death.[xl]

So, what's the take-away from all these sleep studies? What do they ultimately tell us?

Sleep is vital to our physical and emotional well-being. To understand the value of sleep, we must first get a basic understanding of the biological factors which are present and result in sleep and wakefulness. There are two major determinants of wakefulness: our circadian rhythm and homeostatic sleep drive. The circadian rhythm is the reason for our alertness and it varies based on the time of day. It opposes our homeostatic sleep drive (or our "drive to sleep") which is why we have long periods of sleep and can compensate for prolonged wakefulness or strenuous physical activity.

When it comes to the initiation of sleep, melatonin is the key hormone that regulates the sleep/wake cycle. It plays a role in synchronizing the circadian rhythm with the sleep/wake timing. Melatonin is produced by the pineal gland. During the day, the pineal gland is inactive and no melatonin is produced. Once the sun sets and darkness occurs, the pineal gland turns on and produces melatonin. As a result, melatonin levels rise and you feel drowsy and less alert. This results in a desire to sleep. These levels stay elevated in the blood through the night, then fall to low daytime levels once the sun begins to rise. Therefore, light is the dominant factor that controls melatonin. Bright light directly inhibits the release of melatonin. This includes natural and artificial indoor lighting (including lights from artificial devices).

With this basic understanding of how sleep works, the next step is to understand the natural stages of sleep. There are two main types of sleep. One is Non-Rapid Eye Movement sleep (NREM). The other is Rapid Eye Movement sleep (REM). Hang in there with me for a moment as we take a quick look at the four stages of **NREM sleep**.

Stage 1: Slow rolling eye movements and partial relaxation of voluntary muscles. This is defined as a very light stage of sleep. Usually, this is represented as drowsiness to falling asleep.

Stage 2: On an EEG, this stage is defined by K complexes and spindles. This is a deeper form of sleep (though it is still considered light sleep) with increased relaxation. Our heart rate and body temperature go down during this stage. On average, this stage makes up about 50% of our sleep.

Stage 3 & 4: This is the deepest stage of NREM sleep where growth hormones are released, especially in children. During this stage, it becomes difficult to wake the person and it usually occurs in the first third of the night. Your breathing, blood pressure, and body temperature are further reduced during this stage. This stage is crucial for building up your immune function, repairing injured muscle and tissues, and building up energy for the next day.

REM sleep comprises the smallest portion of your sleep cycle. It occurs several times throughout the sleep cycle during the night. It is characterized by the presence of rapid eye movements and is the deepest stage of sleep. Vivid dreaming occurs during REM sleep. Researchers believe this is important for an individual's memory processing and learning. During REM sleep, you have no motor function and experience a loss of muscle tone. In general, there are four to six cycles of NREM sleep per night which are followed by brief intervals of REM sleep. Each sleep cycle lasts about 90 minutes. The percentage of REM sleep tends to be highest during infancy and childhood and decreases as you age. The average adult spends about 20-25% of the night in REM sleep. Most REM sleep occurs in the last third of the night, closer to morning.

THE BENEFITS OF SLEEP

B y now, it should be clear that sleep is necessary and essential to your health. In case you need a little more convincing, let's dig a little deeper into the profound benefits of sleep.

While you slumber, your body is doing some amazing things. Imagine a team of mechanics working to restore your brain, muscles, and organs. This is especially critical for kids and young adults who are actively growing. Real sleep has numerous benefits, some of which we will touch on here.

There's a flip-side to this pillow. If you're regularly deprived of rest, not only do you raise your risk for some chronic health problems, but you may encounter a host of other negative consequences when it comes to your cognitive functioning, such as memory, reaction time, and learning.[xli]

Mental and Brain Health

I'm sure we've all been there. We wake up tired, in a fog, and shuffle through the motions to get dressed and slosh some coffee in a mug. Somehow, we find ourselves at work, but can't remember driving to the office.

A lack of sleep can really tax your brain. Sleep helps your brain work at its best. While you're resting, your brain is getting you ready for the next day. In some ways, it's mending itself from the stresses of the day. For example, new pathways which play a role in learning and remembering information are formed while you sleep.

There's science behind it. Recent studies have shown that a good night's sleep improves learning.[xlii] Sleep also improves your ability to handle problems, big and small. Creativity, decision making, and awareness also improve when you get the proper amount of quality sleep.

The opposite is also true. Lack of sleep can lead to a number of problems, including poor decision-making and consequently, adverse behavior, emotional issues, and even difficulty dealing with everyday life.[xliii] Talk about an accident waiting to happen. You need good sleep to regulate your mood. Of course, we're sure you already know this. This is evident when you or someone you know isn't that pleasant to be around in the morning. Just think about kids that are tired!

There are even more serious reasons why sleep is so important. Lack of proper sleep has also been shown to lead to an increased risk for depression and even suicide. This is especially worrying as it's known to be even more of an issue with our youth.[xliv] Sleep deficient kids are not healthy kids. Lack of sleep in children and teens can cause a myriad of behavioral and mental health issues.[xlv] Sleep deprivation has also demonstrated lower grades and impaired concentration in students.[xlvi] So, get those devices turned off and encourage them to sleep.

The Effects of Sleep on The Body

As we've stated before, sleep allows your body to heal and repair itself, especially your heart and blood vessels.[xlvii] Meanwhile, not sleeping well increases your risk for all sorts of health problems like high blood pressure and heart disease, to name just a few.[xlviii]

A healthy weight is also influenced by good sleep. Studies have shown that losing sleep increases the likelihood of obesity.[xlix] You already know that diet and exercise affect sleep, but consider how poor sleep impacts weight gain, in addition to impairing your athletic performance.

When you sleep, your body maintains a healthy balance of hormones. Ghrelin hormones cause a sensation of hunger, whereas leptin gives you that feeling of being full. When you don't get enough sleep, your ghrelin goes up and your leptin goes down. Ever wonder why you crave that midnight snack? Now you know.

Insulin, the hormone that controls your blood sugar level, is also affected by lack of sleep—raising your risk of diabetes.[l]

Maybe you think a cat nap every now and then can make up for a lack of nightly sleep. Not so fast. Your body thrives on deep sleep. This is especially true with children and teens. Deep sleep causes hormones to be released in your body that promote normal growth while boosting muscle mass.[li] Deep sleep also helps repair cells and tissues, both in children and adults. Furthermore, research has shown that sleep plays an important role in puberty and fertility.[lii]

Do you often find yourself getting sick? That packet of Vitamin C you dissolve into water may not be the fix you need. Your immune system needs good sleep to stay healthy. It will thank you for getting good and regular sleep and, if your immune system is happy, you are much better suited to fight off viruses and other common infections, like the dreaded common cold. In fact, research studies have even revealed that sleep can affect the efficiency of vaccinations. Well-rested recipients of the flu vaccine developed stronger protection against the illness than those who were sleep-deprived and receiving the same vaccine.[liii] When it comes to your health, a good night's rest should be your first line of defense for your immune system during cold and flu season.

You Wouldn't Want Your Airline Pilot Sleepy, Would You?

We've already covered this fact and it shouldn't come as a surprise: those who are sleep-deficient are less productive. Whether it's school or work, sleep-deprived people react slower than those who have gotten a good night's sleep. Imagine if you were an airline pilot, charged with the lives of 300 passengers. I'm sure all 300 would want to know that you got a good night's sleep and your reaction time was spot on.

Lack of sleep can also lead to micro-sleep, those brief moments of sleep that occur when you're normally awake. The danger of micro-sleep is that it happens spontaneously, without your awareness or permission. An example of this would be during a class or while you are at work when you don't remember what actually occurred during a brief period of time. It might be harmless in those scenarios, but now imagine that you're a sleepy pilot or even worse, a passenger on the sleepy pilot's plane. Sleep deficiency, and the micro-sleep episodes that it can cause, can have serious consequences.

Still, many people remain unaware of the dangers of sleep deprivation. Some don't even realize they're sleep deficient. This hazard has been proven repeatedly, from drivers falling asleep at the wheel to boat captains falling asleep at the helm. Sleep deficiency is, in many ways, as dangerous as being intoxicated while driving, easily resulting in accidents and even tragic deaths that could have been avoided.

Motor vehicle accidents aren't the only issue caused by tired people. Whether it's a mistake at work that costs you money or a promotion, a mishap on the factory floor which could result in someone getting seriously injured, or poor school performance, sleep deficiency can manifest in many negative forms. No occasion, endeavor, or occupation is safe from the pitfalls of poor sleep.

And that is why sleep is so important. Sleep helps us think more clearly. It hones our reflexes and sharpens our focus. As sleep researcher Dr. Michael Twery, director of Sleep Medicine, Research and Clinical Research at the National Institute of Health (NIH) put it, "Sleep affects almost every tissue in our bodies. It affects growth and stress hormones, our immune system, appetite, breathing, blood pressure, and cardiovascular health."[liv] For your mind, body, and sanity, please take sleep seriously.

CURRENT SLEEP
RECOMMENDATIONS

By now you may be wondering just how much sleep you should get to stave off all these health risks. Most of us have heard the number eight thrown around. Eight hours of sleep. It's a nice round number. It divides nicely into a 24-hour day, but what do the experts suggest? Let's take a closer look at some of the more current sleep guidelines.

The CDC states that a third of Americans average less than seven hours of sleep a night. A 2007 study looked at British civil servants who reduced their sleep from seven to five hours or fewer a night. Researchers discovered that they were almost twice as likely to die from all causes (especially cardiovascular disease)[lv]. Think about it. If you knew that losing a couple of hours of sleep a night would double your risk of death, would you change your behavior? Would you still give up those sleeping hours to binge watch that show?

You may well ask, how much should I be sleeping? How much should my teenager be sleeping? Recently, the

National Sleep Foundation convened a group of sleep specialists. After their conference, they updated the recommended sleep ranges based on age. Remember, these aren't absolutes that are chiseled-in-stone. Think of them as recommendations based on a consensus of experts.

We do want to stress the importance of sleep for newborns through young adults. Healthy sleep plays a pivotal role in growth hormone release and the development of the brain and body. If you're a parent, pay close attention to the recommendations related to your child's age.

Nightly Sleep Recommendations (in hours)

Newborn (0 - 3 months)	14 - 17
Infant (4 - 11 months)	12 - 15
Toddler (1 - 2 years)	11 - 14
Preschooler (3 - 5 years)	10 - 13
Children (6 - 13 years)	9 - 11
Teenager (14 - 17 years)	8 - 10
Young Adult (18 - 25 years)	7 - 9
Adult (26 - 64 years)	7 - 9
Older Adults (65+)	7 - 8

SLEEP DISTRACTORS

There are three main distractors that can keep us from sleeping: the body, the mind, and the bed. According to the research of Dr. Rubin Naiman, a pioneer in developing integrative approaches to sleep health, these nightly distractions could be stealing your health. Let's take a closer look at each one of these potential distractors and discover what you can do to mitigate them.

The Physical Body

Our bodies are one of the main culprits that keep us from getting the rest we need. There are two main categories we will focus on: what we eat and our exercise.

Nutrition

To start, food and nutrition play a significant role in healthy sleep. Heavy meals should be avoided two to three hours before bedtime. We've all done it. You eat a large satisfying meal right before bedtime and when you try to sleep, you're tossing and turning as your body tries to digest your dinner.

Instead, if you must eat prior to sleep to prevent waking up hungry, consider a small night-time snack with a blend of healthy carbs and protein, such as wheat toast with natural peanut butter or chia seeds with bananas. This should prevent any nighttime hunger.

A frequently asked question is what you should avoid before sleep. There are three common suspects that will steal your sleep: caffeine, nicotine, and alcohol.

Caffeine

Caffeine is a stimulant. It's an adenosine receptor antagonist. That means it blocks adenosine from binding to its receptor. Adenosine plays an important role in your sleep/wake cycle. Because caffeine prevents adenosine from binding to its receptor, it also prevents you from feeling sleepy. A study from 2013 demonstrated that consuming caffeine six hours before bedtime reduced total sleep time by one hour.[lvi] If you love the taste of coffee or tea after dinner, better make it decaf.

Nicotine

Nicotine is also a stimulant and has been shown to disrupt sleep. Research has demonstrated that compared to non-smokers, smokers spend more time in non-REM sleep.

Remember, we need the health benefits of the deeper REM sleep.

Nicotine has also been shown to change sleep architecture, or, in simpler terms, to change the stages of sleep. Multiple studies have shown that smoking has negative effects on overall sleep time, as well as time spent within each sleep stage.[lvii] Regular smokers also take longer to fall asleep. Overall, they spend less time asleep and experience less deep sleep compared to non-smokers. In total, smokers are four times more likely to report feeling unrefreshed after a night's sleep than non-smokers. Quitting tobacco all together will improve your overall sleep quality, as well as provide you with numerous health advantages.

Alcohol

It's not uncommon to have a "nightcap" to finish off a meal. According to the National Sleep Foundation, alcohol is the most commonly ingested substance used as a sleep aid. While it may help you fall asleep, it has actually been shown to suppress REM sleep while also increasing the number of awakenings you will have during your sleep as the alcohol wears off. If you choose to drink alcohol, it's better to drink less, and with a meal.

In terms of diet, if you suffer from gastroesophageal

reflux disease (GERD), try to avoid fatty foods, alcohol, caffeine, and peppermint prior to bedtime. These will make your symptoms worse and possibly prevent you from obtaining good sleep.

When it comes to supporting sleep, magnesium, calcium, and B-Vitamins have been shown to play a role. Before starting any supplements, you should first discuss it with your physician. Our best recommendation would be to avoid caffeine, alcohol, and nicotine six hours before you plan on going to sleep.

EXERCISE

Adequate daytime exercise has been shown to improve sleep. Much has been written regarding the timing of exercise and sleep. Exercise has been shown to decrease stress and "wear you out"—both of which promote sleep. Exercising in the early morning or afternoon also help reset the sleep/wake cycle. Some argue it is best to avoid cardiovascular (aerobic) exercise three to six hours prior to sleep. Some believe, due to the elevation in body temperature by exercise, it may interfere with sleep. This isn't necessarily the case for everyone. Exercise can affect each person differently.

If you find yourself very energized by exercise, you may consider exercising earlier in the day. If it wears you out, try it later in the day. As little as 10 minutes of aerobic exercise, such as walking or cycling, can improve the quality of your nighttime sleep. This is especially true when you exercise on a regular basis.

THE MIND

When we discuss sleep and the mind, we are referring to anxiety, stress, troublesome emotions, and obsessive thoughts. I'm sure you've been there: lying in bed, mind racing, sleep seems fleeting or, even impossible. Fortunately, there are several simple things you can do to overcome your mind and start easing into a restful sleep.

The first step is mitigating stimulus control, or in other words, managing what gets associated with sleep and what doesn't. Unfortunately, when we continue to have restless thoughts and are unable to sleep, we begin to associate our bed and bedroom with those sensations. The goal is to break that cycle and start associating the bedroom with relaxation and sleep. A couple of recommendations to break this cycle are as follows.[lviii]

1. Go to bed only when feeling sleepy

2. Use your bed only for sleep and sexual activity

3. If you can't sleep, get out of bed and do something relaxing until you feel drowsy, then return to bed

4. Get up at the same time every day even if you haven't slept well

5. Don't nap during the day until nighttime sleep improves

There are also pre-sleep practices you can engage in to help prepare for and promote sleep. These include meditation, guided imagery, muscular relaxation, breathing exercises, and gentle yoga. Most importantly, it's a matter of finding a method that works for you and helps promote sleep.

Finally, a personal ritual prior to going to bed is the best way of moving from waking consciousness to a mental state that supports sleep. Some basic examples are journaling, taking a warm bath, a pre-sleep practice, or an activity you find self-nurturing. Any of these can play a role in calming the mind and helping you get into a state where good sleep is obtainable.

THE ENVIRONMENT

Our environment can have a direct impact on the quality of our sleep. Ideally, a bedroom should only be used for sleep and sexual activity. The bedroom should be cool, dark, and quiet. Think of it as a relaxing and peaceful space. Not only should it be clean and comfortable, but it should also feel psychologically safe.

The ideal temperature for sleep has been shown to be 68 degrees or less. Additionally, your bedroom should be a quiet environment. If this is not possible, white noise can be implemented by playing nature sounds, or calming music. In some cases, the sound of a speaking voice has been shown to induce sleep.

The mattress and bedding should be comfortable and free of any toxins, such as pesticides, fire-retardants, or other chemicals. Your mattress and pillow should also provide you with optimal support and comfort.

All clocks should be positioned away from your head. You don't want to be tempted to check the time because this can cause anxiety and promote wakefulness. Approximately 1-3 hours prior to bedtime, start dimming the lights to help induce melatonin production and a sense of sleepiness.

And finally, for ideal sleep, use of any device that emits blue light should be avoided within one hour prior to bedtime. This includes the TV, phone, tablet, or computer. Ideally, there should be no TV in the bedroom. Many sleep-deprived people claim they've sacrificed hours of sleep because of their favorite show.

There are options to purchase blue light glasses, but again, you want to promote the right mental and environmental atmosphere prior to sleep. Reading emails, checking social media, or watching TV doesn't help. On the contrary, those activities can result in a night's worth of ruminative thoughts, resulting in little to no sleep. Our recommandation is to put the electronics outside the bedroom and create a quiet, dark, peaceful environment that allows you to get the rest you need.

Here is another real-life story to consider.

Jill was a female in her 40's who suffered from insomnia. Every night, she attempted to go to bed around 10:30 pm but was unable to fall asleep for at least one to two hours. During this time, she would either lay in bed or got up and worked on her computer to get a jump on the next day.

She drank coffee but did not have a cup after 3 pm. She did not exercise, nor did she have any specific ritual before bed. She would often surf the internet on her phone prior to sleep without the use of any blue light blocking eyewear. Jill was often warm at night, but attributed that to having a warm body.

After some discussion, several recommendations were made. One was to stop looking at any blue screens at least one hour before sleep. The other was to decrease the temperature in her bedroom to 68 degrees at night.

A daily exercise regimen was also recommended. Jill noted she missed yoga and planned to start back up with her daily practice. Another suggestion was for her to begin an evening bedtime ritual, which could include dimming the lights, potentially meditating, or taking a bath before bedtime.

Finally, it was recommended that she not lie awake in bed at night. Instead, she was encouraged to get out of bed and do something (besides work) that could induce sleep. This could include reading a book in a separate room and returning to her bedroom once drowsy. This is important as we want the bedroom to be associated with sleep.

When Jill had the chance to follow up two months later, she reported that she had never slept better and that she was slowly getting back into shape after restarting her yoga practice.

COMMON MYTHS ABOUT SLEEP

The Arizona Center for Integrative Medicine has conducted extensive research into how we sleep, dream, and adapt to sleeplessness. Let's look at some common myths and realities they've discovered about sleep.

Myth: "The mind and body can adapt to less sleep."

Reality: To fully restore itself, the mind and body need to go through all four stages of sleep, particularly deep sleep and REM cycles.

Myth: "We should sleep at least eight hours every night."

Reality: Our personal sleep needs vary with age and other factors. Less than five hours can result in health risks. Ideally, we should get between 7-9 hours.

Myth: "It's ideal to always sleep through the night."

Reality: Occasional awakenings are normal.

Myth: "I can and must make myself sleep."

Reality: We can't control the process of falling asleep.

Myth: "I should just stay in bed and rest if I can't sleep."

Reality: It's best to get out of bed at these times.

Myth: "I'll have a terrible day if I don't sleep well."

Reality: Not necessarily. We are very resilient and can adapt to an off night.

Myth: "Good sleepers fall asleep quickly."

Reality: It's normal to take up to twenty minutes to fall asleep.

Myth: "Good sleepers don't dream."

Reality: Dreaming is an essential part of good sleep.

Myth: "It's best to get up and be productive if I can't sleep."

Reality: Being productive at night can disrupt sleep.

Myth: "It's normal to sleep less as we age."

Reality: It's common, but not inevitable, healthy, or normal.

Myth: "It's comforting to check the time when sleepless."

Reality: Clock watching makes it harder to get back to

sleep.

In Summary

Hopefully, by now, you've discovered some insightful facts about sleep and how it contributes to your health. Let's summarize some key points so you can better prepare yourself for that well-deserved rest.

7 SLEEP STRATEGIES

1) **Ritualize:** Create an energizing ritual with morning light exposure and exercise. Maintain a regular sleep/wake schedule, even on the weekends (don't sleep in for more than one or two hours). Develop a soothing evening ritual as a bridge to sleep.

2) **Use Dusk and Darkness as Sleep Medicine:** Simulate dusk in your home by dimming the lights for a couple of hours before bed. Always use blue light reduction technology to watch TV or when using computers/phones/tablets. Or even better, avoid using those devices completely before bed. Slow down with a warm bath, journaling, rest practices, yoga, or intimacy. Sleep in total darkness.

3) **Watch Your Diet:** Avoid caffeine, nicotine, sugary foods, and adrenaline prior to sleep. Carefully check the possible sleep side effects of all medications you use. Check your alcohol intake, —drink less, earlier, and with food.

4) **Quiet Your Body Noise:** Keep your bedroom cool (68 degrees or less), dark, and quiet during sleep. Keep electric

clocks and other such devices away from your head and bedside. Do all you can to feel psychologically safe in your bedroom.

5) **Learn to Surrender to Sleep:** Avoid the chemical knockout of sleeping pills and alcohol. Approach getting to sleep as a personal spiritual practice, an act of faith. Practice "letting go of waking."

6) **Don't Battle Nighttime Wakefulness:** Go to bed only when you feel sleepy. Never watch the clock from bed, it pulls you back into the waking world. If you can't sleep, get up and sit in a comfortable spot until you're sleepy again. Use nighttime wakefulness as an opportunity.

7) **Arise Mindfully with Intention in the Morning:** Obtain at least twenty minutes of daily exposure to morning light shortly after arising. Awaken slowly and explore your grogginess in the morning. Let the memories of your dreams come and note them. Set conscious intentions to guide your waking day. Use these seven principles to give your body the rest it deserves. Here's to better sleep, a sound mind, and sweet dreams![lix]

MOVE

D o you remember the movie *Wall-E?* If you don't, let me give you a quick refresher on this 2008 Disney-Pixar classic. The year is 2805, and due to pollution, humans have abandoned Earth. The story follows a little robot programmed to clean up the filth humanity has left behind, and for reasons unimportant to this particular synopsis, this little robot ultimately ventures into space where humans now reside in a cruise ship-like spacecraft. Earth's former inhabitants are now all obese and move about in a floating chair-like apparatus. All activities are carried out by simply pressing buttons, and no one walks or even moves for that matter. They rely on these floating chairs to get from point A to point B. In this future, people go through life aided by the inventions they've surrounded themselves with, but ultimately humanity has become a shell of what it used to be.

Although this light-hearted Disney movie intends to be funny, cute, charming, and heartwarming, I found it sobering. I found it sobering because I believe that a technology-assisted, sedentary existence is precisely where we are headed. Unfortunately, we are currently provided more education on how to interact with technology than we are with how to move our bodies. Despite incredible advancements in medicine, we are looking at the first generation in human history to have a shorter life expectancy than their parents.[lx] What if the solution was simple? What if finding the answer depended not on looking to the future, but instead looking backward at the things our ancestors knew. These were what their lives depended on before convenience made existing easy. Specifically, these are the movements that are innate to human function.

This section of *Eat Sleep Move Breathe* focuses on exercise, otherwise known as movement. Our objective is simple: to give you—the reader—practical, applicable exercises you can do to improve your health and wellbeing, starting today. On the topic of exercise, I like to think in terms of what I call boulders and sand. Boulders are the big, non-negotiable (scientifically backed) aspects of why and what. Sand is the tiny minutia that you will find every pseudo-fitness expert arguing about online. To make our agenda crystal clear, we are here for boulders, not sand.

Before you get turned off by the thought of moving rocks, let me explain that I'm not referring to Stonehenge or loading you up with a three hour per day exercise regimen to follow. There are only three boulders, and I call them Why, What, and How. By that I mean: Why exercise is important; What precisely you need to do; How often, and How to perform these movements and routines safely.

WHY DO I NEED TO BREATHE HARD, LIFT WEIGHTS, AND STRETCH?

My three boulders will help build what I like to call "longevity." If you understand these three types of training, why they are essential, and how to properly incorporate them into your exercise regimen, you'll be "cooking with fire," as the saying goes. I mentioned the goal being longevity, which is a concept that's unfamiliar to most. Although many of us understand what fitness or health looks like, most of us rarely consider how health and fitness can affect our freedom. When the aim is longevity, your focus must be on doing that which will support a life unrestricted by the cage that is immobility. This will reduce your odds of developing the preventable chronic diseases that plague our society. In other words, you want a life free from preventable illness. You want to be able to stand without assistance today, tomorrow, and until the day you pass away. It's that simple.

Let us discuss why you need to breathe hard regularly. Researchers have shown that exercise improves your good cholesterol (HDL) while lowering your bad cholesterol

(LDL). They have also demonstrated that exercise strengthens your immune system, increases your lung capacity, and decreases levels of depression and anxiety. And these are just some of the benefits. Biomarkers, or the numbers your doctor rattles off when you go for a check-up (blood pressure and resting heart rate being the most common), are also affected positively by regular exercise. This is particularly true about cardiovascular exercise—exercise that makes you breathe hard for an extended period. It has the unique ability to improve your heart health. If that isn't reason enough to hop on a treadmill and start power walking your way to glory, there has been substantial research in recent years that links this particular type of exercise to significant improvements in mental health, as well.

Fragility in our later years is becoming more and more the norm. As many as one in three women and one in five men over 50 years of age will experience an osteoporotic fracture in their lifetime. According to the Stanford Health Care website, "In individuals with osteoporosis, a fracture can be caused by even a minor fall or during routine activities, such as twisting and bending."[lxi]

In numerous studies, strength training has been shown to improve bone density dramatically. Additionally, there is a strong argument to be made that strength is an essential pre-requisite for nearly every basic human function. Take walking, standing from a seated position, or simply lifting a glass of water to your mouth; each requires a baseline muscular strength to accomplish. While these are all simple tasks that many take for granted, the weaker you are, the closer you are to losing the necessary strength to perform these tasks.

Conversely, the healthier you are, the further away you are from losing those essential functions, and the more prepared you are to perform more complex tasks like running, jumping, or throwing. The best way to think of this is that you are like a fuel gauge. The stronger you are, the closer you are to full; the weaker you are, the closer you are to empty. When your gauge is on empty, you can no longer perform many basic human functions unassisted. Consequently, you must hire human help or, like in the movie *Wall-E*, have machines do those functions for you. When your gauge is full, you not only have the strength to perform these essential human functions with competency, but you also have a solid base for performing other functions not necessary for survival. Instead, these are tasks of choice, like biking, swimming, or more practically, playing a game of tag with your grandchildren.

Let me ask you to try something for me. First, sit on the

ground in the crisscross-applesauce-style you learned in kindergarten. Then, try to stand without using your hands. Were you able to do this? A study completed in 2012, that surveyed over 2,000 adults, showed that this simple test was a predictor of all-cause mortality.[lxii]

What's the catch, you wonder? There isn't one. It's pretty simple—stronger, more mobile people tend to live longer. Just as mobility is a predictor of longevity, like our discussion on strength, many basic human tasks require a baseline mobility. Take the act of sitting down on the couch for example. When Grandma starts to lose the ability to get down to the couch without falling into it or grabbing another object, family members start to become concerned and start discussing the inevitable move to a nursing home. In contrast, when Grandma can perform a full range of motion squat, family members become more concerned that Grandma's much younger boyfriend may not be able to keep up, rather than finding her a caretaker.

HOW TO TRAIN YOUR
CARDIORESPIRATORY SYSTEM

The primary way to train your "cardio" or get you breathing hard, as we called it earlier, is through mono-structural movements. These are cyclical movements that can be continuously performed without rest. Think of exercises like running, rowing, biking, swimming, and skiing.

Recently, we've experienced a rise in the popularity of Functional Fitness programs (F45, P90x, and Orange Theory) to develop "cardio" by utilizing high repetition gymnastics or light weight lifting to produce the same or similar effect. While those exercises can be very effective, they carry a high risk if not performed correctly. If you're interested in that style of training, our recommendation would be to seek a highly trained coach to teach you the intricacies of the techniques so you can perform those movements safely. By whatever means, your objective is a long, sustainable effort that gets you relatively winded.

The easiest and most scalable of all the "cardio" exercises is running—running at ANY speed. If you're a beginner, walking can be a great way to start. There have been multiple studies citing the efficacy of just increasing the number of steps you take in a day as having a dramatic effect on your overall health. When you start to progress, I encourage you not to go from zero to hero. Instead, go from walking to jogging short distances with walking in between. Gradually build the jogging distances longer with shorter walking distances. As an example, a solid year goal for someone starting with no exercise background would be to finish a 5 kilometer (3.2 mile) run without stopping.

The second exercise I want to touch on is rowing. This is a machine that most people shy away from in the gym because they don't know how to use it properly. I'll try to break it down into a few easy steps. Remember the mantra I want you to repeat to yourself through the exercise: "**Legs then arms; arms then legs**."

Rowing

1. Set your feet up in the straps; the strap should hit you about mid-foot

2. Set the damper (tension on the pull) to 5

3. Grab the paddle with a double overhand grip

4. Drive through your feet until your legs are fully extended

5. Pull until the paddle contacts you at the sternum

6. Extend your arms

7. Bend your legs and return to the start position

Like running, start your rowing slowly and build up your endurance and speed over time. A solid one-year goal, coming from an inactive lifestyle, would be to row ten kilometers without stopping.

Strength Training

Strength can be developed in several ways, but ultimately the methodology comes down to utilizing some form of resistance while performing a movement. To build your strength, you can use traditional weightlifting equipment like barbells, dumbbells, and kettlebells, or perform what we refer to as bodyweight movements. There is no need to go and purchase expensive equipment or machines immediately. One item I do suggest buying is a lightweight resistance band for its versatility and practicality, especially for those who travel frequently.

To keep strength training simple, we can break exercise down into four categories or muscle groups: core, back, upper body, and lower body.

You will notice that we have included goals for progress af-
ter a year of adherence to an exercise program. We want to
use these as anchors or targets but to also understand that
progress is largely relative. Give yourself the "ok" to pro-
gress at whatever pace is reasonable. Never lift or perform
something you feel unsafe doing and be proud of every step
you take because ultimately it's further than you have been
before.

Core

The core, for this book's purpose, is defined as the abdominal muscles (six-pack), obliques (meat between your
rib cage and hip), and hip flexors (muscles that cross the
hip). The reason we start with exercises that primarily target
the core is that your success in movements that involve your
arms or legs depends heavily on your ability to stabilize your
core. The simplest and most widely known exercise for your
core is the plank position. There are many variations of the
plank, but we will stick with what's called the low plank.

1. Start with your hands together and arms bent

2. Place your forearms on the ground keeping your hands
   together

3. Straighten your legs out fully behind you

4. Lift your hips and legs from the ground until the only points of contact are your forearms and toes

5. Your body should be in a straight line from the top of your head to the base of your heels

A starting point would be trying to accumulate over three maximal effort holds, a total of 90 seconds in the low plank position. Someone going from completely inactive to active should set the goal of achieving two minutes unbroken after one year of working on this consistently.

Another exercise to add to your repertoire is called the hollow position hold. In explaining this exercise, I will break it down into three separate iterations: beginning level (tuck hold), intermediate level (hollow hold with one leg and one arm extended), and advanced level (full hollow hold).

Beginning Level:

Tuck Hold

* If you are aware of a central hernia or diastasis, do not perform this movement. Rather, strengthen your core through static isometric contractions, such as the plank, NOT abdominal flexion

1. Lay down on your back

2. Squeeze your abdominals as though you were performing a crunch, actively pulling the base of your rib cage down toward your belly button

3. At the top of this movement, your hips and shoulders should be lifted slightly from the ground with the middle of your back being the primary point of contact

4. The top position or hold should have your elbows and knees close together with your hips and shoulders lifted off the ground as mentioned before

Intermediate Level:

Hollow Hold (with one arm and leg fully extended)

1. Lay down on your back

2. Squeeze your abdominals as though you were performing a crunch, actively pulling the base of your rib cage down toward your belly button

3. Extend one arm overhead while holding the other arm across your chest, extend the opposite leg while pulling the other knee up towards your chest

4. In the final hold position, your shoulders and hips should be mostly off the ground with your lower back being the primary point of contact. Additionally, your

extended arm and leg should hover approximately one inch off the ground.

Advanced Level:
Full Hollow Hold

1. Lay down on your back

2. Squeeze your abdominals as though you were performing a crunch, actively pulling the base of your rib cage down toward your belly button

3. Extend both arms overhead and extend both legs out fully, pressing your arms and legs together tightly

4. In the hold position, your shoulders and hips should be lifted off the ground, with the primary point of contact being your mid to low back. Your arms and legs should be approximately one inch off the ground

Your initial objective when starting this regimen should be to hold a hollow position with perfect technique for 90 seconds by the end of your first year. Although the low plank and hollow position hold are certainly not an exhaustive list of core exercises, mastering these two will improve your core strength considerably and move you closer to your fitness goals.

Back

The number one thing that people are concerned about when beginning resistance training is injuring their back. This is for a good reason. Performing lifts without proper mechanics can lead to catastrophic outcomes. With that in mind, the benefits certainly outweigh the potential risks if lifting is performed correctly.

When referring to the back, we are focusing on the spine and its surrounding muscles. The spine is broken down into three basic sections: cervical (neck), thoracic (rib cage and mid-back), and lumbar (lower back). The goal is to strengthen and create awareness in the surrounding muscles on how to simultaneously move and stabilize the spine effectively, or in plain terms, to keep the back safe and get you stronger.

The first exercise I want to cover is called the **sumo deadlift,** due to its transferability to the real world. This movement is essentially the how-to guide on how to pick anything up from the ground to your waist. For that reason, you can use anything to perform it—a backpack, a bag of dog food, one side of a coffee table, or more conventionally a barbell. They are all effective.

1. Straddle the object you are going to pick up in a stance wider than shoulder-width (if this object is a barbell,

walk up to it and place the object about midfoot)

2. Imagine your back is a concrete block as you execute the lift, nothing from your head to your hip should move or change position at all.

3. Hinge at the hip until you reach a position similar to an outfielder in baseball

4. Bend the knees by pushing them out but not forward

5. Firmly grasp the object you are lifting

6. Drive through your legs, with your shoulders and hips rising together until the object reaches the knee

7. Push the hips forward to reach a full standing position

Over a year of work, your goal should be to safely lift an object weighing up to your body weight.

The second exercise is called a **Jefferson Curl**. The goal of this exercise is to increase the awareness of how to move each part of your spine independently.

1. Start in a standing position with your feet under your hips

2. Begin by slowly bending your chin towards your chest

3. Follow that by bending the mid-back forward into flexion as well

4. Go slowly here, vertebrae by vertebrae. Finally, round the lower-back in the same fashion

5. Finish the movement by extending, vertebrae by vertebrae, back up to a full standing position

As stated in the movement's description, the Jefferson Curl should be performed slowly and unloaded. After a year, you should be able to do this movement up to 20 times without needing to rest between repetitions.

Upper Body

When attempting to improve upper body strength, you will need to target three main areas: pushing, pulling, and small muscle stability. With this goal in mind, I will provide a simple exercise designed to kick start your progress for each area.

Pushing

There are many methods you can use to strengthen your pushing power, but arguably, none are more effective than the overhead press. Specifically, we will discuss the seated dumbbell press. It's important to note that when I say dumbbell, I mean two equally weighted objects, and you should not feel limited to using an actual dumbbell. Kettle-bells or even a couple of milk jugs will do if that's all you have available.

1. Start in a seated position on the ground with your legs extended fully in front of you

2. Bring the dumbbells to your shoulders, with one head of the dumbbell resting on your shoulder with your elbows slightly forward from your hands. This position is what is known as the front rack position

3. Press the dumbbells directly overhead extending your arms fully and reaching up as high as possible to support the weight overhead

4. Maintain a stable and neutral position of your body throughout

5. Finish by bending your elbows forward from your hands and bringing the dumbbells straight back down and returning the dumbbells to the rack position

I encourage anyone reading this book to start with light weights to develop great technique, and then incrementally increase your load over time. After about a year, a great goal would be to do three sets of ten with dumbbells totaling a third of your total body weight.

Pulling

For pulling, the **dumbbell row** is a great way to increase your basic strength.

1. Start at a standing position with your arms extended at your waist, grasping the dumbbells

2. Lean forward and hinge at the hip until your torso is close to parallel to the ground (maintain a neutral position of the back)

3. Extend your arms with your palms facing your legs

4. Slowly and deliberately, pull the dumbbells up until they contact you at the base of your rib cage

5. Finish the movement by returning your arms to the starting position

As with the overhead press, start light, master the technique, and build slowly. A good year's goal would be to achieve three sets of ten repetitions with dumbbells totaling one-third of your total body weight.

The last movement, the **banded pull-apart**, is for shoulder stability. It targets the small muscles that help keep your shoulders healthy. If you work at a desk and have become increasingly afraid of becoming the Hunchback of Notre Dame, this exercise will be your best friend!

Along with increasing general stability, the banded pull-apart has an extremely restorative effect and can counteract a lot of the negative side effects people experience when sitting at a computer screen for long hours.

1. Using a light tension exercise band (referenced earlier as the ONLY piece of equipment we'd recommend you shell out cash for) grab one side of the band at shoulder width with your palms facing up while holding the band at chest height

2. Pull your hands apart with slow and steady tension until the band contacts your chest

3. Keeping the tension on the band, slowly return your hands to the starting position

A general rule of thumb with strength building is that the most effective movements are often the simplest. Be skeptical if you need to operate 57 pulleys and a lever to perform the movement on some complex machine. That's probably a good indication that that movement will have little to no application in your daily life. A fair year's goal for this simple and effective banded pull-apart is to perform 40 reps without stopping.

Lower Body

Like the upper body, the lower body can be broken down into three basic movement categories: squatting, jumping, and overall lower body stability.

Squatting

We start with the **squat**. Everyone needs to squat, and if you lose the ability to do so, you will struggle to perform common daily tasks like simply sitting and standing. Over time, the unloaded squat (described below) can also be used to safely perform a squat under load.

1. Start with your feet shoulder-width apart and your toes pointed forward

2. Before beginning the squat, brace by taking a deep abdominal breath and squeezing

3. Start by pushing the hips back

4. Bend the knees out so they track in line with your toes

5. Sink into the squat, getting as low as you can and maintaining proper position of the above points. If anything gets out of position, stop an inch higher and work to that range until it's perfect.

The year goal would be a low (hip crease below the knee) squat maintaining perfect position.

Jumping

The **side-to-side hop** is a wonderful way to increase your balance, coordination, and help with the bone density issue we referenced earlier.

1. Find a crack in the sidewalk or a line on the ground. Preferably, this would be on a firm surface without padding or matting

2. Place both feet together

3. Start by bracing your core, taking a deep abdominal breath and squeezing to stabilize

4. Hop laterally over the line

5. Upon landing, keep your knees in line with your feet and keep your feet together

Note: When you advance, the side-to-side hop can be performed on a single leg as well. At one year, you should look to be able to perform 50 two-footed fluid hops over a line without a break.

Lower Body Stability

The final movement, the **banded sidestep**, targets hip stability and engagement. The hip is arguably the most important joint in lower body function and movement, so strengthening the small stabilizers goes a long way.

1. Take an exercise band and stand at hip distance on one side of the band pulling the remaining side to your waist

2. Take a step with one foot out against the band creating

tension

3. Replace the trailing foot to the same width stance as the starting position

4. Perform the same process on the opposite side

In one year, you should shoot to be able to perform 40 reps on each side without taking a break.

IMPROVE YOUR MOBILITY THROUGH STRETCHING

L ike the previous two sections, this will be a simple guide, not an exhaustive list by any means. The aim here will be to give you a few simple stretches that address large areas and multiple muscle groups. Like the strength section, we will break these down into a few categories, core and back, upper body, and lower body.

The core and back are probably the most difficult group of muscles in the body to stretch. While the **modified triangle pose** that we will cover certainly won't hit every muscle, it goes a long way towards lengthening some of the more difficult and common problem areas.

1. Find a large empty wall space, stand in a straddle stance with your back up against the wall

2. Point one foot forward with the heel up against the wall

3. The other foot should be approximately one foot away, pointing parallel to the wall

4. Lean from the hip toward the foot running parallel to the wall

5. Keeping your back fully against the wall, reach your arm to the foot running parallel

6. As you are leaning down toward the foot, the other arm should stretch overhead toward that side; keep the backs of your arms in contact with the wall throughout

7. Repeat on the other side

You should feel this stretch from the top of your hip, all the way up to your side and into your shoulder. Your aim should be to hold each side for a minimum of one minute without coming out of the stretch.

We talked a bit about the shoulder getting tight from sitting, and especially typing. The **prone shoulder stretch** will help lengthen the muscles that get short and cause pain.

1. Lay on your stomach

2. Reach one arm out to the side, fully extended with your palm down

3. Place your other hand next to your shoulder in the typical pushup position

4. Press into the hand close to your shoulder and rotate your body away from the extended arm until you feel a stretch.

5. Repeat this stretch on the other side

You should feel this stretch in the chest and through the extended arm. You should aim to be able to hold this stretch for one minute on each side.

Are you tired of talking about exercise and working out at this point? How about one more, but it will involve a couch. I knew that would work; enter the couch stretch!

1. Take a couch pillow and place it on the ground, against the base of the couch

2. Place your knee on the couch pillow and your foot on the couch

3. Use the ottoman or coffee table to prop your chest up and put your other leg into a modified lunge position

4. Repeat on the other side

You should feel this stretch in your hip and on the front of your leg. Your aim should be to hold this stretch for one minute on each side.

Now, the big question is how to take all of this and put it into a plan that you can implement tomorrow. Remember, this is a suggested starting point. It is certainly not the only way to do it. What's important is that you start and that you keep going. If you can't handle three days, start with two or one—but start and don't stop.

MY TWO-WEEK PROGRAM

Week One

WEEK 1: DAY 1	Cardio:	Run or Walk 1 Mile
	Strength:	3 sets each 10 seated dumbbell press 10 dumbbell rows 40 banded pull apart
	Stretch:	1:00 min triangle stretch (each side) 1:00 min prone shoulder stretch (each side)

WEEK 1: DAY 2	Cardio:	3 x 500m row 2:00 min rest between efforts
	Strength:	3 sets each 1:00 min hollow hold 10 Jefferson curls 1:00 min plank hold 10 deadlifts
	Stretch:	1:00 min triangle stretch (each side) 1:00 min couch stretch (each side)

WEEK 1: DAY 3	Cardio:	3 x 400m run/walk 1:00 min rest between efforts 3 x 200m run
	Strength:	60 banded side steps in each direction (in as few sets as possible) Then 5 sets 10 unloaded squats 20 side to side hops *rest as needed between sets
	Stretch:	1:00 min couch stretch (each side) 1:00 min triangle stretch (each side)

Week Two

WEEK 2: DAY 1	Cardio:	row 2000m
	Strength:	20 Jefferson curls 4 sets each 10 deadlifts 10 squats
	Stretch:	1:30 min triangle stretch (each side) 1:30 min couch stretch (each side)

WEEK 2: DAY 2	Cardio:	3 x run/walk 800m (rest 6 mins between runs)
	Strength:	4 sets each 1:00 min hollow hold Max plank hold Max banded pull aparts
	Stretch:	1:30 min prone shoulder stretch (each side) 1:30 min triangle stretch (each side)

WEEK 2: DAY 3	Cardio:	5 x 200m run 250m row
	Strength:	Four sets each 20 banded side steps (each direction) 12 dumbbell rows 20 side to side hops 12 seated dumbbell press
	Stretch:	1:30 min prone shoulder stretch (each side) 1:30 min triangle stretch (each side) 1:30 min couch stretch (each side)

As you advance with this program, you can increase the difficulty in several ways. First, you may increase the amount of work by adding rounds or repetitions. Second, you can increase the amount of weight or tension of the band. Finally, you can decrease the amount of rest you take between exercises or repetitions.

> *"Don't be fooled by the calendar. There are only as many days in the year as you make use of. One man gets only a week's value out of a year while another man gets a full year's value out of a week."*
> - Charles Richards

The compounding value that even a light amount of regular exercise will have on your health and fitness is incredible. One thing that's important to consider about longevity is that regardless of how healthy we are, no one knows how much longer we have to live. We have absolutely no control of when we pass away because there are so many uncontrollable factors at play. But we do have control over how we live those days and the quality that marks them. With this, we wish the rest of your days be filled with laughter, play, and unrestricted fun. Movement is key, take it seriously, and you surely won't regret it.

MOVING ON

At eleven, Tony was already overweight and socially withdrawn. The first time I met Tony, he was with his Aunt. He stood there with his back hunched and shoulders slumped. She told me Tony was a great kid, but needed something to help get him active. He was tall for his age, but by the way he stood, all shelled in, he looked like the smallest kid in the class. I reached out to shake his hand, but could tell he didn't want to be here. The gym was the last place he wanted to be.

Over the next year, Tony's routine was to hide in the back of the class and participate as little as possible. He didn't feel like he was fitting in. The less he engaged with the class, the less interest they had in getting to know him.

As a coach, it was hard to watch Tony's behavior. He looked like a kid who was going to give up if we couldn't find a way to better engage with him. One day, we decided to talk to his aunt. We thought it would be a good idea to sign Tony up for a lifting meet our gym was hosting. As Tony shook his head no in the background, his aunt enrolled him for the meet. Tony had regularly attended our lifting classes over the year and had shown great potential. We just needed to get Tony to see what we all saw in him.

On the day of the meet, Tony was set to compete in the deadlift. As he walked in, he had a particularly grumpy look on his face. Not only was he forced to join the gym and the class, now he was stuck in some stupid competition. When Tony started warming up for the deadlift, he looked good—really good. His form looked beautiful. Even though he could easily lift more, the coaches kept the weight light. We didn't want him getting distracted, faltering his technique. When Tony trained, he would do multiple repetitions. But in the weight lifting competition he only had to perform one repetition. That day, Tony's single repetition focus was perfect.

When it was time for Tony's first attempt, he walked onto the platform and lifted 265 pounds with ease. On his second attempt, he lifted 295 pounds gracefully. Now he had everyone's attention. All eyes were on Tony. At thirteen years old, he'd already out-lifted the next best person by 75 pounds. For Tony's final attempt, 315 pounds were loaded onto the bar. A hush went over the room as Tony approached the platform. He grabbed the bar and pulled flawlessly. He stood tall before the roaring crowd. Tony had beat his personal record by over 100 pounds. That moment changed Tony's life.

From then on, he came into the gym with a purpose. He had goals. He had new eating habits. He became more social and outgoing with the other kids. When Tony first joined, he was 5'2" and weighed 225 lb. At age 17, he was 6'1" and 205 lb. That same year, he pulled 525 pounds, setting a state record. Tony is now 21 years-old and remains in regular contact with the coaching staff who helped start him on his path.

The one thing that Tony's journey made me realize is that confidence isn't built overnight. Instead, it comes from taking step after grueling step toward what seems like an impossible peak. Before you know it, you can look back at how far you've come. It's then that you realize your goal is closer than when you started. Confidence doesn't come from thinking you can do it. True confidence comes from knowing the effort you've put into achieving your goal and realizing that if you keep taking the next step, there's nothing that can stop you.

Let today become that first step. Put that first foot forward and focus on getting the next foot moving. Then repeat that process over and over. No matter what road-blocks or detours stand in your way, keep your momentum. Keep moving forward. With the will to move, you are an unstoppable force.

Video Links

Plank:
https://www.youtube.com/watch?v=lOI8pKq8mqE&feature=youtu.be

Hollow Hold:
https://www.youtube.com/watch?v=M6Of_X4Qcoo&feature=youtu.be

Sumo Deadlift:
https://www.youtube.com/watch?v=G0FZz7QPIVs&feature=youtu.be

Jefferson Curl:
https://www.youtube.com/watch?v=dfPWUAXKLmg&feature=youtu.be

Seated Press:
https://www.youtube.com/watch?v=e8PWjO-HAZM&feature=youtu.be

Dumbbell Row:
https://www.youtube.com/watch?v=aKdr5drUbFE&feature=youtu.be

Banded Pull Apart:
https://www.youtube.com/watch?v=WnHEXZP6jBE&feature=youtu.be

Air Squat:
https://www.youtube.com/watch?v=EIJdnPKysfw&feature=youtu.be

Side to Side Hop:
https://www.youtube.com/watch?v=ukcb1bUQJHA&feature=youtu.be

Banded Side Steps:
https://www.youtube.com/watch?v=VoM7hO6ycS0&feature=youtu.be

Triangle Pose:
https://www.youtube.com/watch?v=JvZoRHSiD-4&feature=youtu.be

Prone Shoulder Stretch:
https://www.youtube.com/watch?v=rqshJrH8t80&feature=youtu.be

Couch Stretch:
https://www.youtube.com/watch?v=mEfvCsceCds&feature=youtu.be

BREATHE

Sarah had been isolating at home with her three kids and husband for over three months. Her family noticed she was becoming very irritated and would snap at them for the smallest household infractions. For Sarah, things were stressful. She felt she had no personal space, no time for herself, and just needed to get away. She loved her family dearly but needed a break. Unfortunately, owing to the pandemic, that was not an option.

Sarah's story was all too familiar. It was recommended that she start a meditative practice. The plan was to take at least 10-20 minutes per day, with no distractions, and use a meditation technique of her choice. Sarah found some online meditation guides she could follow and made a rule in her home: when it was time for her meditation, there would be no disruptions. Soon, her family began to see a change in Sarah. Her level of patience and tolerance increased which enabled her to meet the daily challenges of parenting three kids. Her family respected her time and would even announce to visitors, *"Be quiet, Mom is meditating."*

Breathe. Technically speaking, breathe is a verb we use for the process of inhaling and exhaling. However, depending upon the context, "breathe" can be a command to calm down when we're overwhelmed. It can mean to yearn for a sense of freedom as in, "I need a place far away where I can breathe." In what I believe to be its most profound connotation, breathe means to live—as in, "As I live and breathe." In this chapter, we'll discuss mindful breathing—the practice of focusing your attention on your breath, the inhale, and the exhale; these are the basics of meditation.

Many people have the wrong perception of meditation. Some think meditation is the exclusive domain of Buddhist monks, or it's tedious and requires a great deal of patience. In fact, meditation does not require believing in any specific religious tradition and, when practiced daily, has many benefits for your physical and psychological well-being. Your daily routine can be spiritual, non-spiritual, formal, or just a very natural way to start caring for yourself. Meditation simply involves incorporating time into your life where your only focus is on you and not the millions of other things which concern you each day.

We live in a time of constant stimulation. Whether it's

our smartphones, the internet, television, or our friends and family. This ongoing struggle for our attention creates stress, and we know that stress can take a toll over time. You may already suffer from a chronic disease or illness which creates even more anxiety. Meditation can help you find peace in a hectic world, but meditation is designed to be a daily practice, and consistency is critical to producing a desirable result.

We recommend starting a formal meditation practice. If you're not quite there yet, consider incorporating some peace into your daily life. This could be a time that's uninterrupted and allows you to escape the world and your thoughts. It can be as simple as sitting in a park and looking at the trees, or sitting quietly in a peaceful space where you can escape your daily stresses. Where you meditate is up to you, as long as that place provides you some restorative peace. It may help you to know there is no right or wrong when it comes to meditation; it is simply a practice that can help you in your daily approach to life, and allows you to re-energize mentally and spiritually.

WHAT IS MEDITATION?

According to the National Center for Complementary and Integrative Health (NCCIH), meditation is "a mind and body practice that has a long history of use for increasing calmness and physical relaxation, improving psychological balance, coping with illness, and enhancing overall health and well-being."[lxiii] Jon Kabat-Zinn, the founder of the University of Massachusetts Center for Mindfulness, describes meditation as "simplicity itself. It's about stopping and being present. That is all."[lxiv]

In a letter published 10 years ago, the director of the NCCIH wrote that "the literature on meditation suggests that it is a potent tool for learning control of attention, regulating emotion, and increasing self-awareness or cultivation of the state called mindfulness." [lxv] While these insights are well known, scientific data across the last 15 years has shown that during the practice of meditation there are several measurable biological changes, particularly in the autonomic nervous system. Meditation has been clearly shown to have an impact on your mental and physical health. So, even though meditation has been around for centuries, we are just beginning to understand the positive effects it can have on our health.

In the last ten years, there has also been quite a focus on Mindfulness, which is just one aspect of the meditation experience. As defined by Jon Kabat-Zinn, "Mindfulness means paying attention in a particular way; on purpose, in the present moment, and non-judgmentally." The goal of Mindfulness is to have an awareness, moment-by-moment, that disengages you from a strong attachment to beliefs, thoughts, or emotions. The result? Mindfulness creates greater emotional balance, clearer thinking, a heightened sense of compassion, open-heartedness, and well-being. These are results that are good for you and everyone around you and have the added benefit of contributing to a healthy lifestyle.

Why Should I Meditate?

As an individual and a society, we face a daily barrage of stimuli. Many of us suffer from chronic stress, from either psychosocial factors or illnesses which require management tools. Chronic stress can result in increased levels of cortisol, which alone can result in high blood sugar, hypertension, fatigue, and low-grade levels of inflammation which are associated with an increased risk for disease. Many studies have investigated meditation for different conditions, and there's growing evidence that it has multiple health benefits.

Research suggests that meditation can help reduce anxiety and increase positive mental effects. Also, studies have demonstrated that Mindfulness can help prevent depression from recurring. In a 1982 study, Jon Kabat-Zinn demonstrated that chronic pain was reduced when patients were trained in mindfulness-based stress reduction (MBSR).[lxvi]. Studies have also shown that meditation helps with headaches, hypertension, coronary artery disease, overall longevity, cognitive function in older adults, and quitting smoking.

There have also been numerous studies that demonstrate meditation's role in improving symptoms from psychological disorders, including depression and anxiety, and with individuals who suffer from excessive worry. Given these findings, meditation has clearly demonstrated a potential benefit for a wide range of disorders, while also helping you cope with the stresses of daily life.

Health Benefits

One of the primary benefits from meditation appears to be its effect on the autonomic nervous system. This effect results in a decreased sympathetic tone and an increased parasympathetic tone. In simpler terms, all you need to know is that the sympathetic system becomes more active when you are stressed. It is part of the "fight or flight" response.

As the parasympathetic system is stimulated, heart rate and breathing slow, stress hormones decrease, blood vessels dilate, and digestion is facilitated. There have been multiple research studies suggesting meditation can also physically change the brain and body. Gyrification is a brain process in which there is an increase in the folds in the outer layer of the brain. A 2012 study demonstrated gyrification by comparing the brain images of 50 adults who meditated to 50 adults who did not meditate. The study suggested that those who meditate have an increase in folds in the outer layer of the brain which is believed to increase the brain's ability to process information.[lxvii]

Aging is obviously a concern for all of us. We hope to remain as mentally sharp in our later years as we are in our 20's and 30's. A 2013 review of three studies discussed the benefits meditation can have on our normal aging process. It concluded that meditation appears to slow, stall, or even reverse aging-related changes in the brain.[lxviii]

Although research is ongoing, past studies have suggested that meditation can help with a wide range of chronic health conditions, including high blood pressure, psychological distress, anxiety, depression, anger, hostility, and coping ability. Recent studies on meditation's ability to reduce pain have produced mixed results. Even though these studies have demonstrated positive effects on our brain and internal physiology, there is still a significant amount of research needed to learn the extent of the effect meditation may have on our mind, bodies, and aging process.

Mental Benefits

Meditation has also been proposed to have an effect on our emotions. Our emotions are processed in a part of our brain called the amygdala. The amygdala is the area of the brain responsible for emotional responses including interpreting and processing danger and thus plays a central role in anxiety responses to stressful situations. In 2012, the NCCIH set out to determine how meditation might impact this area of the brain. Their study found that different meditation techniques yielded distinct changes to the amygdala's activation suggesting meditation training may effect emotional processing in everyday life, and not just during a meditation.[lxix]

Like many people, you may be thinking about meditation as a way to manage stress and cultivate peace of mind. There are, however, many studies documenting other lesser-known mindfulness meditation benefits which can have a positive impact on mental and emotional health. One study from 2014, a literature review of 47 trials with over 3,000 participants, demonstrated moderate evidence that mindfulness meditation programs could improve anxiety and depression.[lxx]

When it comes to research specifically focusing on meditation and anxiety, a review of 36 trials in 2012 found that 25 of them reported better outcomes (in terms of symptoms) for the meditation group when compared to non-meditation groups.[lxxi]

Meditation can certainly be useful when it comes to mental health though it is important to remember that meditation is not meant to replace conventional care, or to be used as a reason to postpone seeing a health care provider about a medical problem.

Types of Meditation

If you're ready to take some first steps towards starting a daily meditative practice, understand that although there are many types of meditation, most of these have four main elements, according to the NCCIH:

1. A quiet location with as few distractions as possible

2. A specific but comfortable posture (sitting, lying down, walking, or another position)

3. A focus of attention (a specially chosen word or set of words, an object, or the sensations of the breath)

4. An open attitude (letting distractions come and go naturally without judging them)

The more common types of meditation include:

- Transcendental meditation

- Breath awareness meditation

- Zen meditation

- Forest bathing (yes, it's a type of meditation)

- Kriya Yoga

- Walking meditation

- Forgiveness or Metta meditation

Other practices which incorporate a meditative component include yoga and tai chi. In 2017, the National Health Interview Survey found that 14.2% of U.S. adults utilized meditation.[lxxii] Those meditative practices often involved a religious context, though many practice meditation without a specific spiritual focus.

Getting Started

Below you will find two simple techniques to start meditating, as well as a mindfulness exercise you can use daily:

The Basics

1. Find a position of comfort. You can either be sitting or lying down. There are meditation chairs and cushions available to purchase for your comfort.

2. Close your eyes.

3. Breathe. Let it naturally flow in and out. Make no effort to control your breath.

4. Focus your attention on your breath without attempting to control its pace or intensity. Pay attention to the movement of your body as you breathe. This can be as simple as a mental observation of your shoulders, chest, or belly, or watching your breath enter and exit your nose or mouth. If you lose focus or your mind wanders, don't worry, that's normal. Just bring your attention back to your breath. Allow thoughts to simply move through you without paying them any particular attention. Remember, you will get caught in your thoughts. Again, that is normal. Focus less on doing it right and more on continuing to remind yourself to bring your attention back to your breath.

When you start to meditate, practice for two to three

minutes per day. As you become more comfortable with the practice, begin trying to extend your meditations for longer periods.

Mindfulness Practice

A great way to deal with daily stressors is by also starting a mindfulness practice. This can be done briefly, anywhere, and at any time to help you through the moment. The SOAP mnemonic is a great way to remember the steps and get started with this practice. [lxxiii]

Stop: pause, notice your breathing, and settle into the present moment.

Observe: drop into your body, being aware of and feeling whatever is happening at this moment.

Assess: without judgment, recognize the pleasant, unpleasant, neutral nature of this experience and let it go.

Proceed: take a deep breath and move on.

WALKING MEDITATION

The steps below are adapted from a guided walking meditation led by Kabat-Zinn's (2014) *Mindfulness Meditation in Everyday Life and Exercises and Meditations.*

The time required to complete a walking meditation is about ten minutes.

First: Find a location where you can walk about 10-15 paces back and forth. It should be a quiet place where you won't be disturbed. It can be indoors or outdoors, wherever you feel the most comfortable.

Second: Walk along the path you chose while stopping to breathe for as long as you like before returning in the opposite direction. You should pause and breathe at the end of your steps just before turning around. The goal of walking meditation is to focus on walking, which you normally do automatically. You should try to focus on the components of each step:

- Lifting one foot

- Moving the foot a bit forward from where you're standing

- Placing the heel of the foot on the floor first, followed by the rest of the foot

- Shifting your body weight onto the forward leg as the back-heel lifts, while the toes of the foot remain touching the ground

- Lifting the back foot entirely off the ground

- Observing the back foot as it swings forward and lowers

- Paying attention to the back foot as it makes contact with the ground, heel first

- Feeling the weight shift onto that foot as the body moves forward

When it comes to speed, walking meditation should be a slow process that involves taking small, deliberate steps. Steps should feel natural and not exaggerated. Your hands can be clasped together in front or behind you, or hanging at your side, whatever feels comfortable for you.

Third: Your attention should be focused on the sensations you usually take for granted while you are taking steps, such as your breath coming in and going out of your body; the feeling of moving your feet and legs as they touch the ground and move forward; the sensation of your head, neck, shoulders, and back as you utilize them in balancing your body for each step; sounds around you as you take the steps, either from you or from the steps themselves; and finally, whatever your eyes focus on as you are moving across the ground. The goal is to fix your attention on any one of these sensations. If your mind wanders (which it will in the beginning), that's okay. Just notice it wandering and then refocus on one of the sensations.

The more you practice your particular meditation

technique, the more it will bring mindfulness into the rest of your life. You may notice a sense of peace or awareness in other activities you perform. Above all, remember your daily meditation practice is your time. Protect it at all costs and enjoy the peace it can provide. In closing, the following case demonstrates how meditation can be applied to help deal with life's challenges.

Carl was a successful male in his 30's. He was a good friend who had made multiple visits to the ER for chest tightness and palpitations. Each time, he stated he was convinced he was having a heart attack. He had multiple stress tests and visits to the cardiologist, all of whom stated his heart was fine and he was most likely suffering from anxiety.

It took some time, but Carl finally began accepting the fact that maybe it was anxiety. He had a very stressful job and family situation, but otherwise he had no cardiac risk factors, exercised daily, and ate a mostly vegetarian diet.

When he approached me about what to do, I asked him some basic lifestyle questions and encouraged him to continue to exercise as it would also help alleviate some of the stress he may have been experiencing.

When I suggested professional help such as therapy or medication, he expressed strong opinions about not taking medications and felt he could handle his personal issues on his own. That being said, I decided to suggest guided meditations for him to perform daily in an attempt to alleviate his stress. I also suggested a specific breathing technique if he were to have a panic attack. Carl initially rolled his eyes and stated, "I knew you would recommend something like that."

Even though he was reluctant, he started a daily meditative practice, which started with five minutes each morning and each night. Little did I know that five minutes became thirty minutes twice a day. Carl noted he felt calmer than he had in years, though he would still have episodes here and there. During the episodes, he would either meditate or perform the breathing technique which appeared to help. He also shared that he was now considering speaking to a mental health professional, as he felt he had a better grasp of what may be triggering his anxiety.

WELL DONE!

Congratulations! You've not only finished the book, but you're also on your way to starting a new chapter in life. One where you're eating cleaner, feeling rested, having a spring in your step, and maintaining a sounder mind. With a basic understanding of our four pillars of health: Eat, Sleep, Move, Breathe, you have the foundation to build a stronger, healthier you. As you build your future, we'd like to leave you with one last word of encouragement.

What you're practicing is not a diet or exercise routine. Think of it as a new way of life. Like putting on your seatbelt, or tying your shoes, think of these pillars as foundational items that you just do. Make them more than a habit, make them a part of your life.

As you do this, stay positive. The road to a healthier you is full of stress, temptations, and battles. You may not always win each day, but stay positive. Remember to forgive yourself and be resilient. Each choice you make, each step you take toward your health, however small, makes a difference. Remember, improving your health is not an all or nothing approach. Every small step matters.

So why not today? Why not let this day be the start of your journey? You can have a body, mind, and lifestyle that you love but it starts with you making a choice to begin. It starts with a single step. We encourage you to let today be the start of your good health and happiness.

Thank you for letting us be a part of this journey. Here's to a better, stronger you. We salute you. To your health!

ABOUT THE AUTHORS

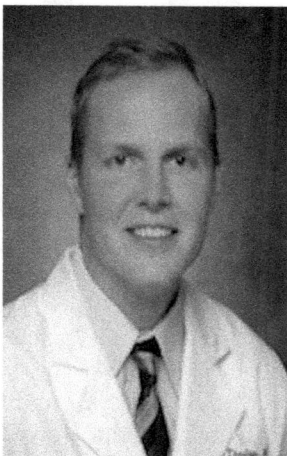

Dr. Lars Thestrup, MD. Dr. Lars Thestrup was born and raised in Northern Virginia where he attended Mary Washington College earning his B.S. in Biology. He received his M.D. at the Medical College of Virginia and completed his emergency medicine residency at Johns Hopkins. Lars then completed a fellowship in North Carolina, focusing on emergency medical services and disaster preparedness at the Carolinas Medical Center. Shortly after the completion of his fellowship, he accepted a position in the City of Houston where he currently serves as an EMS Physician and practices at several emergency departments. Over time, he realized his passion for health and fitness and its role in the prevention of disease which subsequently led him to the University of Arizona Integrative Medicine Fellowship. This has allowed him to continue his journey in helping others evaluate their current lifestyles and assist them in obtaining their individual goals. This book is an extension of that passion which he hopes will transform and educate those truly looking for a change. When he is not working, he loves to spend time outdoors with his wife and two kids.

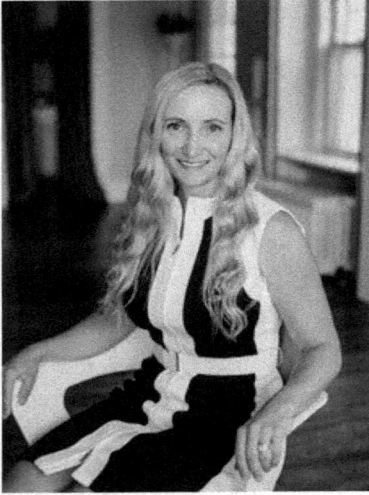

Jennifer Pfleghaar, DO, FACEP, ABOIM.

Dr. Jennifer Pfleghaar was born and raised in Erie, PA. She attended undergraduate at Kent State University with a B.S. in Zoology/Pre-Med and went back to her hometown for medical school at Lake Erie College of Osteopathic Medicine. Dr. Pfleghaar completed her Emergency Medicine residency at St. Vincent Mercy Medical Center in Toledo, OH and a two-year fellowship in Integrative Medicine at the University of Arizona. She works in local community Emergency Rooms around Toledo, OH. She is double board certified in Emergency Medicine and Integrative Medicine. Dr. Pfleghaar is the owner of PflegMed: Center for Integrative Medicine and Natural Aesthetics and Perrysburg Yoga where she sees patients and teaches yoga. Her own health dilemma of Hashimoto's disease, having MTHFR mutations, and having her own children made her journey into Integrative Medicine a passion and a way of life. She lives in Toledo with her husband, Chip, and four children which keep her very busy! They enjoy making gluten/dairy free desserts together and chasing around their backyard chickens.

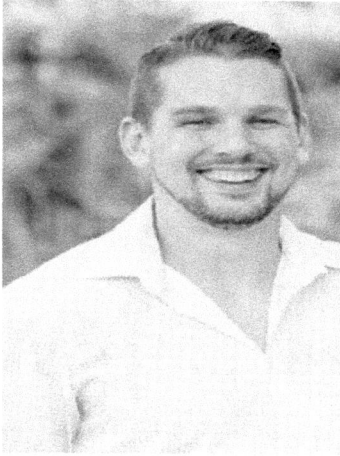

Connor Martin was born in San Diego, California to parents Jeff and Mikki Martin, founders of The Brand X Method, an internationally recognized youth strength and conditioning program. He grew up steeped in the fitness world and is fondly referred to as the "crash test dummy." He is also widely known within the functional fitness community as the original kid participating in this style of exercise. Connor spent his first few adult years as a seminar staff member for CrossFit Inc., teaching the Level 1, Level 2, and CrossFit Kids Seminars to aspiring CrossFit trainers. At the age of 24, Connor moved his young family to Houston, Texas and assumed the head coaching position at CrossFit EaDo and later also CrossFit Central Houston.

Connor is now a lead coach at P3 CrossFit, owns an online fitness company, Compete Elite, and is the International Training Center coordinator for The Brand X Method. He resides in Houston with his fiancé, Michelle, and their three children.

ABOUT
KHARIS PUBLISHING

KHARIS PUBLISHING is an independent, traditional publishing house with a core mission to publish impactful books, and channel proceeds into establishing mini-libraries or resource centers for orphanages in developing countries so these kids will learn to read, dream, and grow. Every time you purchase a book from Kharis Publishing or partner as an author, you are helping give these kids an amazing opportunity to read, dream, and grow. Kharis Publishing is an imprint of Kharis Media LLC. Learn more at **https://www.kharispublishing.com**.

REFERENCES

EAT

[i] Proc Nutr Soc. 2010 Aug;69(3):273-8. doi: 10.1017/S002966511000162X. Epub 2010 Jun 2. Flavonoids as anti-inflammatory agents. Serafini M1, Peluso I, Raguzzini A. Add in 2 Webb AL, McCullough ML. Dietary lignans: potential role in cancer prevention. Nutr Cancer. 2005;51(2):117-31. doi: 10.1207/s15327914nc5102_1. PMID: 15860433.

[ii] Manheimer EW, van Zuuren EJ, Fedorowicz Z, Pijl H. Paleolithic nutrition for metabolic syndrome: systematic review and meta-analysis. Am. J. Clin. Nutr. 102(4):922-32Oct, 2015

[iii] Am J Clin Nutr. 1982 Nov;36(5):873-7. Vegetarianism, dietary fiber, and mortality. Burr ML, Sweetnam PM

[iv] O SS, Yu S, Fedewa A. Systematic review: dietary fibre and FODMAP-restricted diet in the management of constipation and irritable bowel syndrome. Aliment. Pharmacol. Ther. 41(12):1256-70 Jun, 2015

[v] Inflamm Bowel Dis. 2017 Nov.; 23(11):2054-2060. doi: 10.1097/MIB.0000000000001221.

Efficacy of the Autoimmune Protocol Diet for Inflammatory Bowel Disease. Konijeti GG1, Kim N, Lewis JD, Groven S, Chandrasekaran A, Grandhe S, Diamant C, Singh E, Oliveira G, Wang X, Molparia B, Torkamani A.

[vi] Cureus. 2019 Apr 27;11(4): e4556. doi: 10.7759/cureus.4556.Efficacy of the Autoimmune Protocol Diet as Part of a Multi-disciplinary, Supported Lifestyle Intervention for Hashimoto's Thyroiditis. Abbott RD1, Sadowski

A2, Alt AG3.

[vii] Arch Latinoam Nutr. 2008 Dec;58(4):323-9. [Ketogenic diets: additional benefits to the weight loss and unfounded secondary effects].

[viii] Müller H, de Toledo FW, Resch KL. Fasting followed by vegetarian diet in patients with rheumatoid arthritis: a systematic review. *Scand J Rheumatol.* 2001;30(1):1-10. doi:10.1080/030097401750065256

[ix] Pak J Biol Sci. 2012 Mar 1;15(5):255-8. Effect of fasting with two meals on BMI and inflammatory markers of metabolic syndrome. Shariatpanahi MV1, Shariatpanahi ZV, Shahbazi S, Moshtaqi M.

[x] J Pain. 2016 Mar;17(3):275-81. doi: 10.1016/j.jpain.2015.11.002. Epub 2016 Feb 2. Increasing Neuroplasticity to Bolster Chronic Pain Treatment: A Role for Intermittent Fasting and Glucose Administration? Sibille KT1, Bartsch F2, Reddy D3, Fillingim RB3, Keil A4

[xi] Rowe KS, Rowe KJ. Synthetic food coloring and behavior: a dose response effect in a double-blind, placebo-controlled, repeated-measures study. J Pediatr. 1994;125(5 Pt 1):691-698. doi:10.1016/s0022-3476(94)70059-1

[xii,] Arnold LE, Lofthouse N, Hurt E. Artificial food colors and attention-deficit/hyperactivity symptoms: conclusions to dye for. Neurotherapeutics. 2012;9(3):599–609. doi:10.1007/s13311-012-0133-x

[xiii] Stevens LJ, Burgess JR, Stochelski MA, Kuczek T. Amounts of artifical food colors in commonly consumed beverages and potential behavioral implications for consumption in children. Clin Pediatr (Phila). 2014 Feb;53(2):133-40. dio: 10.1177/0009922813502849. Epub

2013 Sep 13. PMID: 24037921.

[xiv] Boris M, Mandel FS. Foods and additives are common causes of the attention deficit hyperactive disorder in children. Ann Allergy. 1994;72(5):462-468.

[xv] Boris M, Mandel FS. Foods and additives are common causes of the attention deficit hyperactive disorder in children. Ann Allergy. 1994;72(5):462-468.

[xvi] The consumption of added sugars (caloric sweeteners) has been linked to obesity, diabetes, and heart disease) Welsh JA, Sharma AJ, Grellinger L, Vos MB. Consumption of added sugars is decreasing in the United States. Am. J. Clin. Nutr. 94(3):726-34 Sep, 2011

[xvii] Joyner, M. A., Gearhardt, A. N., & White, M. A. (2015). Food craving as a mediator between addictive-like eating and problematic eating outcomes. Eating behaviors, 19, 98–101. https://doi.org/10.1016/j.eatbeh.2015.07.005

[xviii] Freeman CR, Zehra A, Ramirez V, Wiers CE, Volkow ND, Wang GJ. Impact of sugar on the body, brain, and behavior. Front Biosci (Landmark Ed). 2018;23:2255-2266. Published 2018 Jun

[xix] Ahmed SH, Guillem K, Vandaele Y. Sugar addiction: pushing the drug-sugar analogy to the limit. Curr Opin Clin Nutr Metab Care. 2013;16(4):434-439. doi:10.1097/MCO.0b013e328361c8b8

[xx] Lenoir M, Serre F, Cantin L, Ahmed SH. Intense sweetness surpasses cocaine reward. PLoS One. 2007;2(8): e698. Published 2007 Aug 1. doi:10.1371/journal. pone.0000698

[xxi] Science. 2019 Mar 22;363(6433):1345-1349. doi: 10.1126/science.aat8515.

High-fructose corn syrup enhances intestinal tumor growth

in mice. Goncalves MD1,2, Lu C3, Tutnauer J1, Hartman TE4, Hwang SK1, Murphy CJ1,5, Pauli C6, Morris R4, Taylor S1, Bosch K7, Yang S8, Wang Y8, Van Riper J8, Lekaye HC9, Roper J10, Kim Y11, Chen Q3, Gross SS3, Rhee KY4, Cantley LC12, Yun J13.

[xxii] Am J Clin Nutr. 2014 Sep;100(3):833-49. doi: 10.3945/ajcn.114.086314. Epub 2014 Aug 6. Fructose, high-fructose corn syrup, sucrose, and nonalcoholic fatty liver disease or indexes of liver health: a systematic review and meta-analysis. Chung M1, Ma J1, Patel K1, Berger S1, Lau J1, Lichtenstein AH1.

[xxiii] Am J Clin Nutr. 2012 Feb;95(2):283-9. doi: 10.3945/ajcn.111.022533. Epub 2011 Dec 28. Sucrose-sweetened beverages increase fat storage in the liver, muscle, and visceral fat depot: a 6-mo randomized intervention study. Maersk M1, Belza A, Stødkilde-Jørgensen H, Ringgaard S, Chabanova E, Thomsen H, Pedersen SB, Astrup A, Richelsen B.

[xxiv] BMJ. 2008 Feb 9;336(7639):309-12. doi:

10.1136/bmj.39449.819271.BE. Epub 2008 Jan 31. Soft drinks, fructose consumption, and the risk of gout in men: prospective cohort study. Choi HK, Curhan G. Soft drinks, fructose consumption, and the risk of gout in men: prospective cohort study. BMJ. 2008 Feb 9;336(7639):309-12. doi: 10.1136/bmj.39449.819271.BE. Epub 2008 Jan 31. PMID: 18244959; PMCID: PMC2234536.

[xxv] Front Biosci (Landmark Ed). 2018 Jun 1;23:2255-2266. Impact of sugar on the body, brain, and behavior. Freeman CR1, Zehra A1, Ramirez V1, Wiers CE2, Volkow ND2, Wang GJ3.

[xxvi] Curr Gastroenterol Rep. 2017 Nov 21;19(12):64. doi:

10.1007/s11894-017-0602-9. The Association Between Artificial Sweeteners and Obesity. Pearlman M1, Obert J2, Casey L3.

xxvii Lippi G, Franchini M, Favaloro EJ, Targher G. Moderate red wine consumption and cardiovascular disease risk: beyond the "French paradox". *Semin Thromb Hemost.* 2010;36(1):59-70. doi:10.1055/s-0030-1248725

xxviii Adv Exp Med Biol. 2017 ; 956 :61-84. doi: 10.1007/5584_2016_147. Impact of Salt Intake on the Pathogenesis and Treatment of Hypertension. Rust P1, Ekmekcioglu C2.

xxix Mayo Clin Proc. 2013 Sep;88(9):987-95. doi: 10.1016/j.mayocp.2013.06.005. Role of dietary salt and potassium intake in cardiovascular health and disease: a review of the evidence. Aaron KJ1, Sanders PW.

xxx Poonamjot Deol, Elena Kozlova, Matthew Valdez, Catherine Ho, Ei-Wen Yang, Holly Richardson, Gwendolyn Gonzalez, Edward Truong, Jack Reid, Joseph Valdez, Jonathan R Deans, Jose Martinez-Lomeli, Jane R Evans, Tao Jiang, Frances M Sladek, Margarita C Curras-Collazo, Dysregulation of Hypothalamic Gene Expression and the Oxytocinergic System by Soybean Oil Diets in Male Mice, Endocrinology,bqz044, https://doi.org/10.1210/endocr/bqz044 Sibille KT1, Bartsch F2, Reddy D3, Fillingim RB3, Keil A4.

SLEEP

xxxi Morris, C. J., Aeschbach D., & Scheer F. A. (2012). Circadian system, sleep and endocrinology. Mol. Cell. *Endocrinolo.*;349;91-104.)

xxxii Ancoli-Israel S., & Rot, T. (1999). Characteristics of insomnia in the united states: Results of the 1991 National Sleep Foundation Survey. I. *Sleep.* 22(Suppl 2): S347-53.

xxxiii Lozoff, B, Wolf, AW, and Davis, NS. Sleep problems seen in pediatric practice. Pediatrics 1985;75:477-483.

Armstrong, KL, Quinn, RA, and Dadds, MR. The sleep patterns of normal children. Med J Aust 1994;161:202-206.

Burnham, MM, Goodlin-Jones, BL, Gaylor, EE, and Anders, TF. Nighttime sleep-wake patterns and self-soothing from birth to one year of age: a longitudinal intervention study. J Child Psychol Psychiatry 2002;43:713-725.

Goodlin-Jones, BL, Burnham, MM, Gaylor, EE, and Anders, TF. Night waking, sleep-wake organization, and self-soothing in the first year of life. J Dev Behav Pediatr 2001;22:226-233.

Mindell, JA. Empirically supported treatments in pediatric psychol- ogy: Bedtime refusal and night wakings in young children. Journal of Pediatric Psychology 1999;24:465-481.

Bixler, EO, Kales, JD, Scharf, MB, Kales, A, and Leo, LA. Inci- dence of sleep disorders in medical practice: A physician survey. Sleep Research 1976;5:62.

Mindell, JA, and Durand, VM. Treatment of childhood sleep disorders: Generalization across disorders and effects on family members. Special issue: Interventions in pediatric psychology. J Ped Psychol 1993;18:731-750.

Byars KC, Yolton K, Rausch J, Lanphear B, Beebe DW. Prevalence, patterns, and persistence of sleep problems in the first 3 years of life. Pediatrics 129(2):e276-84 Feb, 2012

xxxiv National Sleep Foundation's Inaugural Sleep Health Index™. (2014). Sleepfoundation.org

xxxv University of Pennsylvania School of Medicine. (2018, June 5). One in four Americans develop insomnia each year: 75 percent of those with insomnia recover. *ScienceDaily*. Retrieved August 7, 2020 from www.sciencedaily.com/releases/2018/06/180605154114.htm

xxxvi Phillips B, Mannino DM. Do insomnia complaints cause hypertension or cardiovascular disease? J Clin Sleep Med 3(5):489-94 15 Aug, 2007.

xxxvii Institute of Medicine (US) Committee on Sleep Medicine and Research; Colten HR, Altevogt BM, editors. Sleep Disorders and Sleep Deprivation: An Unmet Public Health Problem. Washington (DC): National Academies Press (US); 2006. 3, Extent and Health Consequences of Chronic Sleep Loss and Sleep Disorders.

xxxviii Zimmerman M, McGlinchey JB, Young D, Chelminski I. Diagnosing major depressive disorder I: A psychometric evaluation of the DSM-IV symptom criteria. *J Nerv Ment Dis* 2006;194:158–163.

Schwartz DJ, Kohler WC, Karatinos G. Symptoms of depression in individuals with obstructive sleep apnea may be amenable to treatment with continuous positive airway pressure. *Chest* 2005;128:1304–1306.

Alfano, C. A., & Gamble, A. L. (2009). The Role of Sleep in Childhood Psychiatric Disorders. *Child & youth care forum*, *38*(6), 327–340. https://doi.org/10.1007/s10566-009-9081-y

xxxix Yaggi HK, Concato J, Kernan WN, Lichtman JH,

Mohsenin V. Obstructive Sleep apnea as a risk factor for stroke and death. NEJM 2005;353(19):2034-2041.

Bradley TD, Logan AG, Kimoff RJ, Series F, Morrison D, Ferguson K, Belenkie I, Pfeifer M, Fleetham J, Hanly P, Smilovitch M, Tomlinson G, Floras JS. Continuous positive airway pressure for central sleep apnea and heart failure. NEJM. 2005;353(19):2025-2033.

Caples SM, Gami AS, Somers VK. Obstructive sleep apnea. Annals of Internal Medicine. 20015;142(3):187-197.

Liu Y, Tanaka H. Fukuoka Heart Study Group. Overtime work, insufficient sleep, and risk of non-fatal acute myocardial infarction in Japanese men. Occupational and Environmental Medicine. 2002;59(7):447-451.

Ayas NT, White DP, Manson JE, Stampfer MJ, Speizer FE., Malhotra A, Hu FB. A prospective study of sleep duration and coronary heart disease in women. Archives of Internal Medicine. 2003;163(2):205-209.

[xl] Kripke DF, Garfinkel L, Wingard DL, Klauber MR, Marler MR. Mortality associated with sleep duration and insomnia. Archives in General Psychiatry. 2002;59(2):131-136.

Tamakoshi A, Ohno Y. JACC Study Group. Self-reported sleep duration as a predictor of all-cause mortality: Results from the JACC study, Japan. Sleep. 2004;27(1):51-54.

Patel SR, Ayas NT, Malhotra MR, White DP, Schernhammer ES, Speizer FE, Stampfer MJ, Hu FB. A prospective study of sleep duration and mortality risk in women. Sleep. 2004;27(3):440-444.

[xli] Waterhouse, J. Circadian Rhytms in Cognition. Progress in Brain Research. 2010;185:131-153.

Frenda S,F enn, KM. Sleep less, think worse: The effect of sleep deprivation on working memory. Journal of applied Research in Memory and Cognition. 2016;5(4):463-469.

Alhola, P., & Polo-Kantola, P. (2007). Sleep deprivation: Impact on cognitive performance. *Neuropsychiatric disease and treatment*, 3(5), 553–567.

[xlii] *Maria Bagby (25 February 2014). "The Role of Sleep in Memory, Learning, and Health". Therapeutic Literacy Center. Retrieved 29 September 2018.* "To understand the big picture, give it time – and sleep". *EurekAlert.* 20 April 2007. Retrieved 23 April 2007.

Tononi, Giulio; Cirelli, Chiara (1 January 2006). "Sleep function and synaptic homeostasis". *Sleep Medicine Reviews.* **10** (1):49–62. doi:10.1016/j.smrv.2005.05.002. Graves L, Pack A, Abel T. Sleep and memory: a molecular perspective. Trends Neurosci. 2001;24:237–43. [PubMed] [Google Scholar]

Maquet P. The role of sleep in learning and memory. Science. 2001;294:1048–52[PubMed] [Google Scholar]. Stickgold R. Sleep-dependent memory consolidation. Nature. 2005;437:1272–8.

[PubMed] [Google Scholar].

Ellenbogen JM, Hulbert JC, Stickgold R, Dinges DF, Thompson-Schill SL. Interfering with theories of sleep and memory: sleep, declarative memory, and associative interference. Curr Biol. 2006;16:1290–4.[PubMed] [Google Scholar].

Walker MP, Stickgold R. Sleep, memory, and plasticity. Annu Rev Psychol. 2006;57:139–66.

155

Killgore WDS. Effects of sleep deprivation on cognition. Prog Brain Res 185: 105–129, 2010

xliii Watling J, Pawlik B, Scott K, Booth S, Short MA. Sleep loss and affective functioning: more than just mood. Behave Sleep Med. 2017;15(5):394–409. doi: 10.1080/15402002.2016.1141770.

Brown LK. Can sleep deprivation studies explain why human adults sleep? Curr Opin Pulm Med 18: 541–545, 2012.

Vandekerckhove M, Cluydts R. The emotional brain and sleep: an intimate relationship. Sleep Med Rev 14: 219–226, 2010 [PubMed] [Google Scholar]

xliv Zimmerman M, McGlinchey JB, Young D, Chelminski I. Diagnosing major depressive disorder I: A psychometric evaluation of the DSM-IV symptom criteria. *J Nerv Ment Dis*2006;194:158–163.

Schwartz DJ, Kohler WC, Karatinos G. Symptoms of depression in individuals with obstructive sleep apnea may be amenable to treatment with continuous positive airway pressure. *Chest* 2005;128:1304–1306.

Fawcett J, Scheftner WA, Fogg L, Clark DC, Young MA, Hedeker D, Gibbons R. Time-related predictors of suicide in major affective disorder. Am J Psychiatry. 1990 Sep;147(9):1189–94. doi: 10.1176/ajp.147.9.1189. [PubMed] [CrossRef] [Google Scholar]

Ağargün MY, Kara H, Solmaz M. Sleep disturbances and suicidal behavior in patients with major depression. J Clin Psychiatry. 1997Jun;58(6):249–51. [PubMed] [Google Scholar]

Turvey CL, Conwell Y, Jones MP, Phillips C, Simonsick E, Pearson JL, Wallace R. Risk factors for late-life suicide: a prospective, community-based study. Am J Geriatr Psychiatry. 2002;10(4):398–406.

xlv Cara A. Palmer, Candice A. Alfano. **Sleep and emotion regulation: An organizing, integrative review.** *Sleep Medicine Reviews*, 2016; DOI: 10.1016/j.smrv.2015.12.006

xlvi Roth, Daphne Ari-Even; Kishon-Rabin, Liat; Hildesheimer, Minka; Karni, Avi (1 February 2005). "A latent consolidation phase in auditory identification learning: Time in the awake state is sufficient". *Learning & Memory.* **12** (2): 159–164.

xlvii McAlpine, C.S., Kiss, M.G., Rattik, S. *et al.*Sleep modulates haematopoiesis and protects against atherosclerosis. *Nature* 566, 383–387 (2019).

xlviii Kasasbeh E, Chi DS, Krishnaswamy G. Inflammatory aspects of sleep apnea and their cardiovascular consequences. *South Med J*2006;99:58–67.

Calhoun DA, Harding SM. Sleep and Hypertension. CHEST 2010;138(2)434-43.

xlix Beccuti, G., & Pannain, S. (2011). Sleep and obesity. *Current opinion in clinical nutrition and metabolic care, 14*(4), 402–412.

Taheri S. The link between short sleep duration and obesity: We should recommend more sleep to prevent obesity. *Arch Dis Child* 2006;91:881–884.

Morselli L, Leproult R, Balbo M, Spiegel K. Role of sleep duration in the regulation of glucose metabolism and appetite. Best Pract Res Clin Endocrinol Metab. 2010;24:687–702.[PMC free article] [PubMed] [Google Scholar]

Knutson KL. Sleep duration and cardiometabolic risk: a review of the epidemiologic evidence. Best Pract Res Clin Endocrinol Metab. 2010;24:731–743.

[l] Mesarwi, O., Polak, J., Jun, J., & Polotsky, V. Y. (2013). Sleep disorders and the development of insulin resistance and obesity. *Endocrinology and metabolism clinics of North America*, *42*(3), 617–634.

Beccuti, G., & Pannain, S. (2011). Sleep and obesity. *Current opinion in clinical nutrition and metabolic care*, *14*(4), 402–412.

Gottlieb DJ, Punjabi NM, Newman AB, Resnick HE, Redline S, Baldwin CM, Nieto FJ. Association of sleep time with diabetes mellitus and impaired glucose tolerance. Archives of Internal Medicine. 2005;165(8):863-867.

Knutson KL, Ryden AM, Mander VA, Van Cauter E. Role of sleep duration and quality in the risk and severity of type 2 diabetes mellitus. *Arch Intern Med* 2006;166:1768–1764.

[li] Ritsche, K., Nindl, B. C., & Wideman, L. (2014). Exercise-Induced growth hormone during acute sleep deprivation. *Physiological reports*, *2*(10), e12166.

[lii] Lateef, O. M., & Akintubosun, M. O. (2020). Sleep and Reproductive Health. *Journal of circadian rhythms*, *18*, 1. https://doi.org/10.5334/jcr.190

N. D. Shaw, J. P. Butler, S. M. McKinney, S. A. Nelson, J. M. Ellenbogen, J. E. Hall. **Insights into Puberty: The Relationship between Sleep Stages and Pulsatile LH Secretion**. *Journal of Clinical Endocrinology & Metabolism*, 2012; DOI: 10.1210/jc.2012-2692

[liii] Taylor, D. J., Kelly, K., Kohut, M. L., & Song, K. S. Is Insomnia a Risk Factor for Decreased Influenza Vaccine Response?. *Behavioral sleep medicine*,2017; *15*(4), 270–287.

Spiegel K, Sheridan, JF, Van Cauter, E. Effect of Sleep

Deprivation on Response to Immunization. JAMA. 2002;288(12)1471-1472

[liv] The Benefits of Slumber. NIH News in Health. https://newsinhealth.nih.gov/2013/04/benefits-slumber. April 2013.

[lv] Ferrie J, Shipley M, Cappuccio F, Bruner E, Miller M, Kumari M, Marmot M. A Prospective Study of Change in Sleep Duration: Associations with Mortality in the Whitehall II Cohort. Sleep. 2007;30(12): 1659-166

[lvi] Drake C, Roehrs T, Shambroom J, Roth, T. 2013. Caffeine Effects on Sleep Taken 0,3, or 6 hours before going to bed. Journal of Clinical Sleep Medicine. http://dx.doi.org/10.5664/jcsm.3170).

[lvii] Jaehne A, Loessl B, Barkai Z, Riemann D, Hornyak M. Effects of nicotine on sleep during consumption, withdrawal, and replacement therapy. Sleep Med Rev. 2009;13(5):363-377.

Caviness M, Anderson, B, Stein, M. Impact of Nicotine and Other stimulants on Sleep in Young Adults. Journal of Addiction Med. 2019;13(3):209-214)

[lviii] Hauri, P, Shirley, L.*No More Sleepless Nights*. New York City, NY. John Wiley &Sons; 1996

[lix] Adapted from "7 Strategies for Serene Sleep." Arizona Integrative Medicine Fellowship Syllabus, 2014.

MOVE

[lx] Olshansky, S., Al., E., Preston, S., Baker, M. G., Boulware, D. R., & Cavalcanti, A. B.,et al. (2005). A potential decline in life expectancy in the United States in the 21st century:

NEJM.

[lxi] Standford Healthcare. Osteoporotic Fractures. (2019, December). https://stanfordhealthcare.org/medical-conditions/back-neck-and-spine/osteoporotic-fractures.html

[lxii] O Barbosa Barreto de Brito, L., Rabelo Ricardo, D., Sardinha Mendes Soares de Arau´jo, D., Santos Ramo, P., Myers, J., & Gil Soares de Arau´jo, C. (2012). Ability to sit and rise from the floor as a predictor of all-cause mortality. *European Journal of Preventive Cardiology.*

BREATHE

[lxiii] Meditation in Depth. National Center for Complimentary and Integrative Medicine. https://www.nccih.nih.gov/health/meditation-in-depth. April 2014.

[lxiv] Rakel, D. *Integrative Medicine 4th Edition.* Philadelphia, PA: Elsevier; 2017.

[lxv] Briggs, J. (2010) Letter from the Director NCCIH, National Center for Complimentary and Integrative Medicine. https://www.nccih.nih.gov.

[lxvi] Kabat-Zinn, J. An outpatient Program in behavrioral medicine for chronic pain patients based on the practice of mindfulness meditation: theoretical considerations and preliminary results. *General Hospital Psychiatry.*1982; 4(1): 33-47.

[lxvii] Luders E, Kurth F, Mayer EA, et al. The unique brain anatomy of meditation practitioners: alterations in cortical gyrification. *Frontiers in Human Neuroscience.* 2012;6:1–9.

[lxviii] Luders E. Exploring age-related brain degeneration in meditation practitioners. *Annals of the New York Academy of*

Sciences. 2013;1307:82–88.

lxix Desbordes G, Negi LT, Pace TW, et al. Effects of mindful attention and compassion meditation training on amygdala response to emotional stimuli in an ordinary, non-meditative state. *Frontiers in Human Neuroscience.* 2012;6:1–15.

lxx Goyal M, Singh S, Sibinga EM, et al. Meditation programs for psychological stress and well-being: a systematic review and meta-analysis. *JAMA Internal Medicine.* 2014;174(3):357–368.

lxxi Chen KW, Berger CC, Manheimer E, et al. Meditative therapies for reducing anxiety: a systematic review and meta-analysis of randomized controlled trials. *Depression and Anxiety.* 2012;29(7):545–562

lxxii Clarke TC, Barnes PM, Black LI, Stussman BJ, Nahin RL. Use of yoga, meditation, and chiropractors among U.S. adults aged 18 and older. NCHS Data Brief, no 325. Hyattsville, MD: National Center for Health Statistics. 2018.

lxxiii Rakel, D. Integrative Medicine 4th Edition. Philadelphia, PA: Elsevier;2017

www.ingramcontent.com/pod-product-compliance
Lightning Source LLC
Chambersburg PA
CBHW071236290326
41931CB00038B/3107